AN EDGAR CAYCE HOME MEDICINE GUIDE

Introduction by
Gladys Davis Turner

Printed in the U.S.A.

CONTENTS

INTRODUCTION

In the concepts of health and healing in the Edgar Cayce readings, two principles predominate, imbuing all else that is stated or implied. One is that the health of the body, mind, and soul are so closely interrelated that it is rarely of value to treat any one of these aspects without also giving some attention to the state of the other two. The second premise is that, for every human ill, remedies can be found in nature in the abundance of herbs, fruit, seeds and creatures with which the earth has been endowed. Of this first principle of wholeness much has been written, primarily in reference to the mental and spiritual aspects. The second is the subject of this book.

All of the Edgar Cayce physical readings, with few exceptions, were given for individuals with different needs. This probably explains why there is often slight variation in formula, dosage, manner of application, etc., even between readings on the same subject. Certain products, herbs, oils and formulas, however, were recommended so repeatedly and emphatically that they have become almost specifics for certain types of disorders.

The Edgar Cayce readings, however, should not be viewed as a do-it-yourself doctoring manual. *Any of these suggestions in treatment of disease should be used under the supervision of a professional.*

A.R.E.'s Health Care Professionals Program includes doctors (M.D.s, osteopaths, chiropractors), physical and massage therapists, licensed psychologists, psychiatric social workers and nurses—all A.R.E. members who have agreed to treat clients according to the readings. To use their services A.R.E. members borrow a Circulating File* on a particular ailment and request the names of referred professionals in their locality. The particular member then determines the kind of treatment required and contacts the professional who will help him/her carry out the treatment.

Some of these health care professionals are attempting to study *all* readings given for individuals suffering with a particular disease. In this way a pattern of treatment may evolve which can be tested and the results made public. Some of these reports appear bi-monthly in *The A.R.E. Journal,* taken from Dr. William A. McGarey's monthly "Medical Research Bulletin," all of which are shared annually at the A.R.E. Medical Symposium in Phoenix, Arizona, sponsored by the A.R.E. Clinic, Inc., the Edgar Cayce Foundation and Atlantic University.

The quotes in this book are all taken out of context; hence, the constant reminder to see the entire Circulating File (CF).* Even the CF, however, in most instances presents only a cross section from the many readings that might have been given on an ailment. Thus it is imperative that your own health care professional** study all of the material available and, after diagnosing your condition, prescribe the suitable methods to follow.

The Edgar Cayce Handbook for Health Through Drugless Therapy, written by Dr. Harold Reilly and Ruth Brod, is occasionally referenced throughout this book where applicable.

So often in the Edgar Cayce readings a patient was told, "Either do all of these or none at all!" It is your own physician who should plan a regime for you which may or may not include various methods suggested in Edgar Cayce's readings for the individuals long ago. That is, some of the recommendations for those other individuals *may not apply to you!* Hence the appearance of warnings throughout the book.

Credit for compilation and research of material in this volume is due to the Heritage Store staff in cooperation with the A.R.E. editorial staff and the Edgar Cayce Foundation.

Gladys Davis Turner

---

*Circulating Files are collections of verbatim readings and readings extracts selected and arranged by topic. An ongoing research program is constantly adding new subjects to the current collection. Files are available on loan to A.R.E. members. The current list of medical Circulating Files can be found in the Appendix of this book.

**A list of Health Care Professionals in your area is available to A.R.E. members by request from the A.R.E. Membership Department. For membership information write A.R.E., Box 595, Virginia Beach, VA 23451.

ACIGEST

Acigest was a 10% hydrochloric acid solution with each c.c. containing 11.88 mg. of potassium iodide. This was recommended as a digestive aid and was always to be taken in raw milk. Since certified raw milk cannot be purchased in most states, making Acigest has become impractical. As of 1976, however, Humco Laboratories was manufacturing a 10% hydrochloric acid solution available as an over-the-counter drug.

ACNE SCAR MASSAGE [528-2]

This particular formula was recommended in a reading for a case involving acne *scars*. It is not advised for everyone, although its popularity indicates that it may be effective in some types of active cases.

The ingredients are camphorated olive oil, witch hazel and Nujol (equivalent to Russian White Oil). The formula is an antiseptic and an astringent, recommended "For the exterior forces where abrasions have left the effects, especially. . .scar tissue, where the eruptions show. . ." Prior to the use of the lotion, the reading advised gently scraping the skin "when the tissue forms into eruptions and collects (the matter in same). . ." with a piece of glass or pottery. This "would be much better than any prick or the like, and will cleanse the skin more thoroughly. Then. . .massage. . ." (528-2)

For more information on origin and treatment of skin disorders, consult the CFs on Acne and Complexion.

ADIRON

This product was originally known as Codiron. Adiron was recommended in about 30 readings, particularly for anemia, poor assimilations and general debilitation. It contained cod liver oil and was a source of vitamins A, B, D, E and G. In 1941

Adiron was manufactured by Lawrence Labs in Chicago, Illinois. The readings found that Adiron would supply energy to the body, preventing colds and congestion and reducing tendencies toward infection. White's Codliver Oil tablets are a possible substitute.

AL-CAROID

Al-Caroid is an antacid compound recommended in about 180 readings for acidity, incoordination between assimilations and eliminations, poor digestion, and toxemia, and for related problems such as poor assimilations, poor eliminations, and flatulence. It was also suggested in several cases of cholecystitis, or inflammation of the gall bladder.

This product is still on the market, but only in tablet form and not in the powder preferred by the readings. Additionally, the manufacturers report that the Al-Caroid formula was altered in 1969 to increase its acid-neutralizing effect. One reading suggested Bisodol as an alternative.

ALPINE RAY/RINO RAY

These terms were brand names for sunlamps. The Alpine Ray was a mercury quartz lamp made by the Hanovia Chemical Company in Newark, New Jersey. Since the Alpine and Rino Rays were recommended interchangeably at least once, it seems possible that they were of the same type. Another brand of sunlamp or natural sunlight, when obtainable, might be substituted for these appliances.

ANTI-NAUSEA FORMULA

This was a typical version of formulations recommended primarily in cases of nausea, including seasickness, carsickness, baby care, and nausea due to pregnancy. It was also sometimes indicated in digestive disturbances. This product was manufactured for several years but has been discontinued due to insufficient demand.

The formula contained limewater, cinnamon water, iodide of potassium and bromide of potassium. About a fourth of the approximately 90 readings recommending it did not include the iodide and bromide of potassium in the formula. The limewater and cinnamon water were intended to react with the gastric juices, having eliminant and sedative properties, while the potassiums were intended to act on the nerve impulses. The nausea remedy was to be made fresh by a druggist, who would add each ingredient *in the order named* for each occasion of use, and not to be kept on the shelf for any length of time. See pertinent CFs for more information

ARTHRITIS MASSAGE FORMULA [3363-1]

Massage was frequently advised in cases of arthritis, as a valuable portion of the treatment regimen. One formula that is widely used was described in reading 3363-1. The ingredients are: Nujol, olive oil, peanut oil, oil of pine needles, sassafras oil, and lanolin, and include those most often suggested for arthritis massage.

Peanut oil was the single most frequently suggested massage oil, both by itself and in combination with other oils. The readings claim that:

Those who would take a peanut oil rub each week need never fear arthritis. **1158-31**

And [using] the [peanut] oil rubs once a week, ye will never have rheumatism nor those concurrent conditions from stalemate in liver and kidney activities. **1206-13**

A combination of peanut oil and olive oil was often recommended, with variants such as the addition of pine needle oil and lanolin.

. . .olive oil—properly prepared (hence pure olive oil should always be used)—is one of the most effective agents for stimulating muscular activity, or mucous membrane activity that may be applied to a body. **440-3**

Oil of pine needles was an ingredient in about 25 arthritis massage formulas and sassafras oil was also included in about ten of these compounds, so that many similar massage combinations for arthritis exist in the readings. Many of these formulas could probably also be used in other instances requiring massage. Such formulas, containing oil of pine needles and sassafras oil, have been prescribed for a wide variety of complaints, including paralysis, impaired locomotion, multiple sclerosis, Parkinson's disease, spinal subluxations, neuritis, debilitation (weakness), injuries, and nervous problems. Other oils commonly used in such formulas are oil of wintergreen and cedarwood oil.

In another reading the following comments were made regarding a formula that is similar to the Arthritis Massage Formula with the exception of sassafras oil:

Also each week (on the same day each week) we would have a thorough oil rub, to stimulate all the activities of the glandular centers, or coordinating centers in glandular patches and lymph patches along the spine with the cerebrospinal and sympathetic nerve centers.   3304-1

Use of the Arthritis Massage Formula should follow an Epsom salts bath. Epsom salts is commonly prescribed in inflammatory afflictions of this type.

For more information consult the CF on Arthritis or other appropriate files. (See also Dr. Harold Reilly's book, *Handbook for Health Through Drugless Therapy,* detailing "Cayce Massage Mixtures.")

ATHLETE'S FOOT REMEDY [291-1]

The external treatment for athlete's foot most commonly used from the readings is derived from reading 291-1. The formula contains Nujol, witch hazel, sassafras oil, and pure kerosene, and this combination is apparently a very effective fungicide.

To massage same [affected areas] with this preparation would be well (as it would be for any).   291-1

See CF on Athlete's Foot.

ATOMIDINE

Atomidine is "atomic iodine," valuable because it is iodine in a form apparently less toxic to the body than the molecular iodine generally available in kelp tablets, or Lugol's Solution. For this reason the approximately 610 Cayce readings that mention Atomidine are enthusiastic about its usage in cases involving glandular deficiency or malfunction associated with a shortage of iodine in the system. Atomidine was recommended for a wide range of illnesses, and in readings on the subject, the Cayce source stated:

4

. . .this may be used for the dental, the hygiene, and the internal—*wherever* there is an indication of an unbalancing of either the gland or the assimilating and eliminating system activity. . .   358-1

This will not only be a curative property, but a *preventative!* May be used internally and externally as well, and especially for any form of disorder in glands *or* tissue of body.   358-2

The readings further stated that Atomidine ". . .will purify the glandular system so as to resist adverse influences. . ." (1521-2)

We would add then, in specifics, those elements that will increase the flow of secretions or activities in the glands of the system (as related to the ductless), and as to the blood supply for stimulation; which would be found in the compound known as Atomidine.   411-1

Though Atomidine is a safe external remedy for anyone, it should be used internally with care—and legally is a prescription item when used internally, because of its high iodine content. It can be harmful to anyone who takes too large a dosage. *Each drop of Atomidine supplies approximately six times the minimum daily requirement of iodine.* Too much iodine can lead to overstimulation of the thyroid gland, resulting in nervousness, insomnia, and rapid heartbeat. Even a skin rash can result from too much iodine taken over a period of time. The few readings which warned about taking too much Atomidine, however, were for individuals who were already deriving sufficient iodine from other sources, such as Calcios, Calcidin, or diet. Atomidine should not be taken at the same time as other iodine-containing drugs, including those mentioned above, as well as the Formula from 636-1, kelp tablets, and any multiple vitamin or mineral tablet containing iodine.

Atomidine was rarely prescribed as a treatment by itself, but was to be used as a part of various programs, also involving other important measures. One of its uses is in some cases of baldness, where internal dosages of Atomidine supplement external application of crude oil. Atomidine was also recommended in cases of arthritis (internal application), feminine hygiene, prevention of splitting fingernails (internal and external application), poison ivy (internal and external), goitre (internal), leukemia (internal), venereal disease (external), prevention of infantile paralysis (internal and external), asthma (internal), dental care (internal and external), use as a gargle (diluted) for sore throat, and use as external application for cuts, boils and surface infections.

For more precise details on dosage and application of Atomidine,* consult the appropriate CFs.

BALSAM OF SULPHUR

This was a liniment recommended about 35 times in the readings, often for such conditions as paralysis, impaired locomotion resulting from arthritis, and misplaced vertebrae. Two different types of treatments were suggested. The one most often mentioned involved massaging about a handful of the balsam over the cerebrospinal system. The other treatment was to massage this liniment over the lympth gland areas, including the armpits, neck, abdomen and groin. In both treatments, properties from the balsam are absorbed by the body, and as with other massage solutions only the amount which the body will absorb should be used. A few minutes after the massage the body was to be washed off with a weak solution of bicarbonate of soda, made in the proportion of one teaspoonful to a gallon of water. The readings generally suggested that this massage be given three to four times weekly or every other day, and often recommended that it precede or follow a spinal adjustment.

Instructions for preparing the balsam of sulphur are as follows: Boil sulphur and linseed oil together in the proportion of one pound of sulphur for each pound of linseed oil. Boil until the resulting combination is "not too wet or too dry," but can be held in the hand.

Extreme caution is advised, as the boiling mixture is exothermic—that is, it can easily explode or catch fire. A double boiler or a water bath may be used.

B-BATTERY

The B-Battery or Dry Cell was the readings' term for an electrical appliance mentioned about 40 times. It was often recommended as a substitute for the Wet Cell* and occasionally for the Radio-Active Appliance,* when no one was available who could make them. Conditions in which it was mentioned

---

*It is recommended that you consult a physician before using this product.

included nervous strain and impaired locomotion.

The B-Battery was based on an ordinary dry cell battery with two positive poles, one carrying 45 volts and the other 22½. It was used just as the Wet Cell is used, with two wires, the same plates, a solution jar, and a lead jar cathode. The battery was available in most hardware stores in the 1930s and '40s.

Edelmann's Ionizer (just called the B-Battery in the readings) was the above battery with a rheostat attached to reduce the current flow to a volt or a fraction of a volt. Edelmann was a New York City manufacturer, and his battery and rheostat were available in many drugstores at the time. What it was popularly used for is unknown.

Unlike most electrical appliances, the useful life of this battery is apparently quite limited. Cayce instructed users to throw it away after 40 days of treatment and buy a new one. It is not known whether the proper type of battery can still be found.

BENZOSOL

Benzosol is an old term for guaiacol benzoate, which contained close to equal parts of benzoic acid and guaiacol. It was sometimes mentioned as an inhalant ingredient and at times as an ingredient in capsules to be taken internally for its stimulating effect on the respiration.

BISODOL

This product was recommended in about 20 readings for the relief of acid indigestion and its accompanying symptoms, such as flatulence, fullness and headache. In one reading Bisodol was suggested as a substitute for Al-Caroid, an antacid that is no longer on the market in the powder form which the reading recommended.

The powder form of Bisodol, which was characteristically mentioned in the readings, has been in existence since 1927. Its active ingredients are sodium bicarbonate—a mild alkali used for relief of hyperacidity of the stomach, and magnesium carbonate—an antacid and laxative. The tablets do not contain the same ingredients. Neither of the Bisodol formulations are exactly the same as in Cayce's day, as all antacids were modified to conform to rules and regulations published in the Federal Register in June of 1974. However, according to the makers of Bisodol, there have been no major changes in the formula since it was first marketed.

A notation from Gladys Davis: I keep Bisodol on hand and use it occasionally, with good results, for the symptoms indicated on the label.

See the CF on Indigestion and Gastritis.

BLACK & WHITE PRODUCTS

The Cayce readings seldom referred to specific Black & White products, although the brand in general was recommended frequently. [811] was advised to use Black & White cosmetic aids in preference to the cosmetics she was then using, because "these are more beneficial to the cuticle [skin]." (811-4) Another reading stated that "the Genuine Black & White products are nearer to normal." (2072-6) They are recommended, at least in part, for their alkalinity:

As to the face lotion, we find that a cream that is less acid will be the more beneficial. A test of these may be easily made before they are used. Both the red and blue litmus test are the better way for testing same. And any that is wholly alkaline and non-acid is preferable. The Black & White, as we have indicated, is excellent. 275-37

Another reading claimed these preparations to be "preferable to most of the compounds that carry leads or poisonous conditions for the skin." (2154-2)

The Cold Cream, Cleansing Cream and Vanishing Cream may be used in the same manner as are other preparations of similar cosmetic nature. The Ointment is useful in cases of acne and minor skin rashes. The Skin Whitener may be used to lighten dark spots on the skin. The readings comment further on the effect of these preparations on the skin:

The Black & White are the better preparations for keeping muscles, or the whole body, or the face, in the proper condition. 3051-3

As a cleansing cream and the healing properties for the face and neck, use the *Genuine* Black & White products. These as we find will purify and give a stimulation and a food value to the pores of the skin itself to assist in the conditions already produced, until the *general* health and conditions aid in adjusting same. 2175-2

Whether the Black & White products are the same now as

they were in 1925-1944 when recommended in the readings is impossible to tell. The readings often specified the *Genuine* Black & White made in Chicago, and not Plough's, which is located in another part of the country. Plough's, however, is the maker of the present Black & White products, and claims that it has always been their sole manufacturer. According to Plough's, some of the products once bore a Chicago label because of a warehouse located there. Some of the labels at present do include the word "Genuine."

For more information consult the CF on Complexion.

BODY POWDER

In about 50 readings a special kind of talcum powder was recommended, containing tolu or Peruvian balsam and zinc stearate. Both of these active ingredients are known for their healing properties, and at the time the readings recommended them, were ingredients in a powder manufactured by Johnson & Johnson, which has since gone off the market.

The powder was prescribed to help soothe irritations arising from skin rashes. The majority of these cases are described as dermatitis, and about one third of the readings under this heading were given for babies. It was also mentioned in cases of acne, eczema, pruritus (itching), psoriasis and shingles.

A reading given for a two-month-old baby stated that it "will keep down these disturbances from heat." (2781-1) A reading for a two-year-old found that it "will relieve the itching. . ." (5520-6) The following is a typical comment on this subject:

Should there continue to be the irritation of the skin, use some good powder—as stearate of zinc powder—with balsam. Use this for the rash that occurs on parts of the body.   69-6

For more information consult the Baby Care CF and appropriate files indexed under Skin, such as Dermatitis and Pruritus.

BONCILLA PACKS

The Boncilla packs were referred to about eight times in the Cayce readings. The main ingredient of this preparation is a special type of clay, which was recommended in one reading on the basis of its chalk content:

As we find, the Boncilla would be more preferable than this [another brand of mud pack], that is more of the nature of chalk in same.

1709-5

The packs function primarily as an astringent. After being applied damp to the face, the clay begins to dry and contract, shrinking the pores and tissues of the skin, and resulting in a stimulating, refreshing feeling. The packs bring an increased circulation to the areas to which they are applied. Sometimes this manner of treatment was found helpful for persons with imperfect complexions, as in the following reading:

For the deep-seated conditions [blackheads], the body would find it well to use the mud packs on face and neck—Boncilla— with the oil rubs, then, following same. We would find, we would eliminate the accumulations under the skin without bruising it, and bring a great deal better conditions for the body.

2072-16

For the "oil rubs" to follow the pack, peanut oil, olive oil, or a combination such as in Massage Formula [1968-7] would be suggested.

Another reading implies that possible skin disturbances following an initial application of the Boncilla pack should be regarded as part of an adjustment process toward greater normalcy:

Of course, the mud packs will be beneficial; the first time these would apparently give a great deal of disturbance, but after that the reaction will be much better. Give these for self, you see, and we will find better conditions for the whole of the complexion, as well as the general health of the body. 1709-4

Once or twice a month is generally sufficient for application of the Boncilla packs.

For more information, consult the CF on Complexion. This product is currently not available.

CALAMUS OIL

Calamus oil is of herbal derivation and was recommended as a massage ingredient in at least nine readings involving a variety of cases, which included arteriosclerosis, aftereffects of birth injuries, epilepsy, neuritis, paralysis, Simmonds' disease and spinal subluxations. It was prescribed in a reading involving cataracts in a massage formula combining calamus oil, olive oil and tincture of myrrh to follow osteopathic corrections.

For more information consult the appropriate CF.

CALCIDIN

Calcidin is primarily a source of calcium and available iodine in tablet form. The readings' occasional mention of the "salt" it contains probably refers to calcium iodate. The manufacturers claim that the Calcidin formulation has not changed since Cayce's day, when it received recommendations in about 130 readings. Sometimes Calcidin was prescribed for lung problems, particularly for asthma and tuberculosis, and also in some cases of cold and congestion, coughs, and bronchitis.

The effect of Calcidin on the lungs was described as follows:

The salt and iodine combined in the proportions as they are in Calcidin are to act with the mucomembranes of the lungs themselves, so that there is more oxygen inhaled in same taken into the blood supply through same.   294-166

Calcidin is available in one-grain tablets, and dosage suggested in the readings varies from one grain daily to as many as five grains every few hours if needed, in cases such as asthma. The manufacturers advise taking each dosage with half a glass of hot water, and the readings sometimes added the suggestion that the tablet(s) be taken dissolved in the water.

Asthma:

To assist the lungs, the bronchials, the larynx, to overcome that asthmatic condition as appears from time to time, use tablets (five grain) [of] Calcidin, see? Let these dissolve and swallow same, as they dissolve in the mouth, see? or this may be dissolved and taken as a dose, or it may be taken internally, see? This will reduce the irritation. These may be taken every few hours, when it's necessary, but, as the manipulation and the adjustments are made, these may be gradually reduced, as the diet is kept with same, and we will build the system. . .90-1

. . .these [tendencies to wheeze], during this period when the complete adjustments are being made, should be aided with the combining in the system—taken internally—those of Calcidin, that will add both calcium and iodine to the system in sufficient quantity and manner as to gradually *lose* these

impulses and influences in the body. We would take these regularly, in one two-grain tablet each day, and when a spasm of the reaction should occur, these we would dissolve in hot water and take—which will be found to bring relief almost immediately, provided the rest of the system is kept in a nominal attitude [normal condition].   3738-1

Q-1. Should I continue to take adrenalin?
A-1. As we find, it would be much better to change to the other climate and to take Calcidin. . .   5004-1

Tuberculosis:

Then in the application of the Calcidin for the throat and the pressure upon the lungs: To be sure, this may be overdone; that is, there may be made to be too great an iodine reaction in the system.
Hence, while this should be kept ready, it should be altered in its application so that it is only used when *necessary,* see?
                                                                 1045-10

When, and *if* the body goes to the higher climate or higher altitude, or a more even climate, take Calcidin; in this manner: Dissolve three to five grains of the Calcidin in an ounce of distilled water; keep this warm, and once or twice a day sip about half a teaspoonful. *Do not* take this, though, in the low altitude—or close to the seashore; for the effect of the iodine in the circulation would not be as efficacious in the low altitude as in the high. . .
Do not take calcium separate, for you will get sufficient in the Calcidin—which is calcium and iodine in combination—that works with the system in such conditions.   1560-1

Hence, we would occasionally have the activity of Calcidin; one grain taken once or twice a day will be most beneficial. Not so much as to have the reaction from the iodine, save as secondary; but the combination of the calcium and the iodine upon the system will stimulate the circulatory forces as related to the general circulation. . .
Then the influences to purify the blood supply (the calcium, with the iodine), also those for the lungs through the use of the inhalations [from charred oak keg] indicated, will tend to so build resistance as to prevent this [tuberculosis] becoming an activative force in the bloodstream.   289-8

Cold and Congestion:

In [the] present condition Calcidin should be taken of an evening, or when there is lowest resistance in [the] system, or when congestion is the greatest. Should be taken in two-and-a-half- or three-grain tablets, or may be dissolved in water and sipped occasionally when irritation in the throat is disturbing. Should be taken in small quantities. Best in this liquid form.   137-129

Q-2. Should the doses of Atomidine* be continued?
A-2. We would leave these off in the present; for the Caldicin carries sufficient of the iodine reacting principle—if those properties are given in the manner indicated. . .   1521-4

Cough:

For the immediate future there has been sufficient of the iodine and calcium (Calcidin) for the system, though this has aided much in giving the proper balance in the activity of the thyroid, the proper balance in the digestive forces as related to the character, the quality, the kind of assimilated forces by this increase. . .
Occasionally, if there is the cough that makes for a great disturbance in the evening or night, a grain of the Calcidin may be taken. It will aid in producing rest for the body.1110-4

As mentioned in the above reading, Calcidin, because of its iodine content, also influences the endocrine glands, particularly the thyroid:

[Take Calcidin] that there may be the reaction not only of the iodine upon the glands of the system but also of the calcium for *its* assimilation through not only the digestive forces but through the circulatory forces—as it is absorbed more by this sipping *through* the circulatory forces of the body. This will aid in keeping down the temperature, aid in making for a helpfulness through the lungs, and add to the activity of the glands themselves throughout the system.
Glandular *strain* and the *lack* of the necessary influences in the system to supply activity through the glands [are indicated by the condition of the body—tumors and dry skin]. Hence the iodine *and* the calcium in the system (through the taking of the Calcidin as indicated) will supply these chemical elements to aid, and hence will reduce the *possibility* of these becoming of a tumorous nature. For if the system is balanced in its chemical reaction, these things disappear. It will also aid in the lung tissue as well as in the activities of the spleen, the pancreas and the gall duct.   954-2

---

*It is recommended that you consult a physician before using this product.

The addition of the iodine and calcium (in the Calcidin) will not only aid in creating a better circulation for the teeth, the gums and mouth, but—if a grain of this is dissolved in water and the gums *and* the mouth rinsed with same, it will not only aid the teeth and the eyes but all the gland forces of the body!

263-20

See appropriate CFs. It is recommended that you consult a physician before using this product.

Gladys Davis added the following information: Calcidin was recently discontinued by its manufacturers. I am sorry about this because many, including myself, received help through its use when needed for the symptoms on the label.

CALCIOS

Calcios was recommended in about 200 readings. In the 1930s and '40s it was made from pulverized chicken bones, processed so that the calcium it contained could be easily assimilated and digested. Calcios was the calcium supplement that the readings invariably recommended.

The cases in which Calcios was most often prescribed in the readings (percentages approximate) were tuberculosis, 20%; poor assimilations, 15%; pregnancy, 10% and glands, 5%; comprising a total of 50% of the instances in which Calcios was mentioned.

Following is a composite of several statements from the readings on Calcios for some of the cases listed above:

Tuberculosis:
[1548] was told there was free calcium available in Calcios, and that it strengthened the blood by making the covering of the blood cells stronger. [1569] was told it contained a necessary force for body building. [2168]'s reading said that tuberculosis germs were present in the body, but that Calcios would prevent them from becoming destructive forces.

Assimilations:
Calcios contains the digestive enzymes pancreatin, pepsin, and hydrochloric acid. [1792] was told that through the use of Calcios the assimilations would be greatly improved.

Pregnancy:
It is well known that pregnant women have a high calcium requirement. [951] was told, "Calcios is the better manner to

take calcium. It is more easily assimilated, and will act better with pregnancy than any type of calcium products as yet presented [on the market.]" (951-7) She was told to have a whole wheat cracker spread with Calcios three times weekly at the noon meal until two weeks before the baby was due. To [73] the readings advised Calcios rather than calcium tablets, as it would be better assimilated and not be too hard on the liver and kidneys. [480] was told it would be good for the baby's bones and would replace that drained from the mother.

Arthritis:
For a young man crippled with arthritis this advice was given:

Calcium is now needed, in a manner that it may be assimilated, and gradually take the place of that which has been crystallized in the bursa and portions of the structural body. This we would add in the form *which we have indicated as the BEST*—the chewing of bones or ends of bones of the fowl [bony pieces of chicken, well stewed, until soft]. If this is abhorrent to the body, or disagreeable, then take Calcios, about three times each week, just what would cover a Premium cracker as butter. Best that this be taken of evenings.
849-43

CAMPHORATED OLIVE OIL

The ingredient consistent in most of the readings which referred to a treatment for scars is camphorated oil, either alone or in combination with other oils. Readings 440-3, 1208-3 and 566-3 state that camphorated oil should be prepared from camphor and olive oil rather than the commercially available camphorated cottonseed oil. The following reading describes the effects of the camphorated olive oil on the skin:

Olive oil—properly prepared (hence pure olive oil should always be used)—is one of the most effective agents for stimulating muscular activity, or mucous membrane activity, that may be applied to a body...
The camphorated oil is merely the same basic force [olive oil] to which has been added properties of camphor in more or less its raw or original state than the spirits of same. Such activity in the epidermis is not only to produce soothing to affected areas, but to stimulate the circulation in such effectual ways and manners as to combine with the other properties in bringing what will be determined, in the course of two to two and a half years, a new skin! **440-3**

For old scars, undiluted camphorated oil may be used. In treatment of recently formed scars the readings suggest dilution of the camphorated oil with substances such as cocoa butter, compound tincture of benzoin, peanut oil, lanolin, and olive oil itself. The purpose of this dilution is to avoid "burning" the scarred area, and the amount of dilution would depend on the tenderness of the scarred areas. The diluted camphorated oil should be gently rubbed once daily well into the areas affected, preferably just around the edges of the scarred area rather than directly onto the scars themselves. This should prevent the formation of permanent scar tissue and allow the normal healing process to occur:

. . .we would massage the body—not so much over the area itself but *along* the sides of same and over those areas from which this portion of the body receives its impulse for circulation to the superficial portions of the body—with camphorated oil. 1165-1

If he wants to relieve much of the scar tissue on the left limb, we would use sweet oil [olive oil] combined with camphorated oil (equal parts). Massage this each day for three to six months and we would reduce most of this. 487-15

In a case of burns, camphorated oil was prescribed "to prevent or remove scars, as the tissue heals." (2015-6)

Complete healing of old scars should be expected to require months or even years of consistent treatment, "but remember the whole surface may be entirely changed if this is done persistently and consistently." (440-3)

In the approximately 80 readings in which camphorated oil was recommended, it was also given other uses, particularly in cases of cold and congestion:

First we would massage as much camphorated oil in the spine, chest and throat, as the body will take up. 324-1

Then, be sure that the body is massaged well with camphorated oil between the shoulders and around [the] throat, between the eyes and around the head and the places where there is the soft tissue in [the] face—all that it will absorb. . .

Well that in the evenings before retiring, for the next two days, the feet be bathed in hot water and then rub them well to the knees with the camphorated oil also. 415-3

Keep the [camphorated oil] rubs for the body, as it will assist in strengthening the spine and aid the development of the structural portions of the body.

The massaging across the chest, around the ribs, also aids in the circulation for more and better blood.   1200-6

In 566-3 the camphorated olive oil was recommended for massage in combination with equal parts of mutton suet, spirits of turpentine and spirits of camphor:

The variation in the camphorated oil (which is, of course, camphor added to olive oil) will make for an opening to the pores of the body, you see.   566-3

For more information, consult the CFs on Colds and Scars.

CAROID AND BILE SALTS
(Now Caroid Laxative)

Caroid and Bile Salts was the name of a laxative compound recommended in about 90 readings. The active ingredients were caroid, a digestive aid; capsicum, a mild gastric stimulant; bile salts, or salts of the bile acids; phenolphthalein, which has laxative properties; and cascara sagrada, a mildly laxative herb. This compound was intended to improve the digestion of proteins, increase the flow of bile enabling the body to more properly handle fats in the diet, and effectively and gently relieve constipation. In the Cayce readings, Caroid and Bile Salts was recommended primarily in cases of poor eliminations, incoordination between assimilations and eliminations, and toxemia:

. . .these [properties] are the active principles that function with the gastric forces of the duodenum and the liver itself, in producing functioning with the gall duct itself, supplying the stimuli and—when supplying the stimuli—necessarily drawing *from* the system the energies in other portions of the body.   359-2

. . .for these should cleanse the system and aid in draining the gall duct area, lessening this pressure upon the liver and the *causes* from same as produced by the engorgement in the colon.   1141-1

Q-1. What can be done about stiffness in fingers?
A-1. Increase the eliminations as indicated; first by the

adjustments so that drainages are set up nominally, and then by the period of eliminations [so] that when there are the reactions from the organ's activity in the alimentary canal the drainages will be naturally from the superficial circulation to the other portions or organs of activity in the eliminating system. 389-7

These will be for producing an activity to the functioning of the excretory or secretive activities of the liver, the spleen, the pancreas. 1057-1

Q-1. Just how many and how often should the Bile Salts be given?
A-1. Until they remove the condition! 265-13

Caroid and Bile Salts was often recommended in combination with Al-Caroid:

In the present we would find that the better applications would be to use the Al-Caroid as a digestant and as an eliminator of the acid in the system, used with the Caroid and Bile Salts as an eliminant and as an active force with the liver and digestive system. 265-8

These will *cleanse* the whole system. 985-1

The Al-Caroid and Caroid and Bile Salts were sometimes to be taken alternately and sometimes on the same days. Reading 2051-1 advised that they be taken together in periods of two to three days, alternated with two to three rest days. Caroid and Bile Salts, as with most laxatives, were not to be taken indefinitely:

These are of such natures that you will come to depend upon them. Hence if the treatments suggested are taken, gradually leave off the tablets. 3574-1

Caroid Laxative tablets have evolved from the original Caroid and Bile Salts recommended in about 90 readings. As a result of the over-the-counter drug review in which the FDA laxative panel concluded that laxatives should not contain non-laxative ingredients, the formula now contains only two of the original five active ingredients: phenolphthalein, a chemical having laxative properties, and cascara sagrada, a laxative herb.

Unfortunately, the new Caroid Laxative no longer offers

such a wide spectrum of benefits. Lacking the ingredients which aided the digestion, it is now only a laxative, although probably still a good one.

As with all preparations of this type, Caroid Laxative should not be taken indefinitely, as this can lead to dependence on laxatives. The readings suggested that their use be gradually discontinued, as other treatments followed at the same time began to have their normalizing effects.

For more information, consult the CFs on Intestines: Constipation; and Stomach: Indigestion.

CARRON OIL

Carron oil was a liniment consisting of equal parts of lime-water and linseed oil, also known as "lime liniment." It was first made in Carron, Scotland, where it was found useful for treating burns received by workers in the Carron ironworks.

This compound was a massage ingredient in three readings. In one instance the reading stated that carron oil, along with the other ingredients combined with it, would aid in increasing circulation along the spine:

> The ingredients are of such a nature that the properties will strike *into* the activities of the lymph and the bursa circulation around each of the ganglia along the cerebrospinal system, if massaged in a rotary motion from the head to the middle. . .
>
> 585-3

Carron oil was mentioned in one reading for a case of detached retina. In speaking of the condition in the retina of [679]'s right eye, the Cayce source commented that if the proper adjustments and massages were given, the eye would return to normal:

> This in the body, as we find, is produced by conditions in the upper dorsal and in the cervical area by the accumulations, and is *not* in itself of a local condition! As we make these applications [massage] and these adjustments, and the blood flow is increased, these conditions should clear up. . . 679-1

For more information, consult the CF on Eyes: Detached Retina.

CASTILE-BASED SOAP AND COCONUT OIL SOAP

Castile soap is a variety of soap based on or containing olive oil or other vegetable oils, and was mentioned about five times in the readings. Apparently the reason for these recommendations is its gentleness to the skin. A reading for a baby advised:

Do not use a soap in the bath that is caustic! for this makes for irritations to the new skin! 1208-5

When asked what soap would be best, the reply was: "Castile; pure." (1208-5)

Q-5. What soap. . .would be least harmful and most helpful in correcting and beautifying the skin?
A-5. Pure castile soap is the better as a cleanser. 2072-6

Obviously, choice of soap is an individual matter, and castile was one among several deserving enough to be termed in one reading as "any good soap. . ." (1968-7)

Coconut oil soap was mentioned in one known reading. For this individual at least, soap made with either coconut oil or olive oil was found preferable to those based on other kinds of fat or oil.

See CF on Complexion.

CASTOR OIL

Another name for castor oil is Palma Christi, or palm of Christ. It seems appropriate that a plant with such a name should historically be used in healing, although the readings did not customarily endorse using it in the same manner—as a powerful cathartic—as many of us were forced into during childhood.

It should be noted that there were a few cases in which internal dosage was recommended, while other readings strongly cautioned against it. In general, less drastic means of cleansing the intestines were preferred:

Castor oil taken internally, and such eliminants are only purgatives. Hence the castor oil absorbed from the packs will be better than taking same internally. 1433-6

In contrast, castor oil has a great variety of external uses. A mixture of castor oil and baking soda was advised for application on callouses on the feet, moles, ingrown toenails and warts:

Apply a paste of baking soda with castor oil. Mix together and apply of evenings. Just the proportions so it makes almost a *gum;* not as dough but more as gum, see? A pinch between the fingers with three to four drops in the palm of the hand, and this worked together and then placed on—bound on. It may make for irritation after the second or third application, but leave it off for one evening and then apply the next—and it will be disappearing. 1179-3

In about 50 additional readings castor oil was recommended for use in massage, including application for callouses, cancer (skin and breast), cysts, bunions, moles, tumors and warts. The use of castor oil in the form of packs, however, was advised most frequently, in about 570 readings. The packs were indicated most often for cholecystitis (inflammation of the gall bladder), poor eliminations, epilepsy (for which they were almost a specific), various liver conditions such as cirrhosis and torpid liver, and scleroderma; and also for headaches, appendicitis, arthritis, incoordination between assimilations and eliminations, colitis, intestinal disorders such as stricture and colon impaction, incoordination between nervous systems, neuritis, and toxemia.

The following readings offer typical instructions for use of the packs:

Heat the oil; dipping two, three to four layers of flannel in same, wring out and apply directly to the body. Well that dry heat [heating pad] be kept over same during the period of an hour or the like when the packs are on the body. Bathe off the body afterwards, of course, with a weak [baking] soda solution, to cleanse the body from the acidity and from the natural secretions that arise from same 1034-1

Be well to put oil paper or cloth [or plastic] over the packs, for we should have great quantities of the oil. Do not make them *too* hot, but so as to at least drive them into the body. It is well to put these on and then apply external heat; as the electric pad or salt bags or the like. *Dry* heat, though, rather than wet heat. 1312-3

The castor oil packs may be continued daily, applying for several hours at a time if necessary, until relief is obtained; or, they may be taken according to a cycle, such as three days of using the packs alternated with four rest days. The taking of olive oil in combination with the packs is often advised. Reading 2521-1 suggests: "Following the third castor oil pack, at the end of the third day, you see—give internally two table-spoonsful of olive oil."

Reading 1553-7 comments that "we will find it will work well with the assimilating, and act as a food as well as an eliminant for the alimentary canal."

Do not attempt to use the apple diet as a cleanser, if using the [castor] oil packs.   543-27

Often the heavy or woolen flannel was specified. In some cases, a colonic irrigation was recommended following a series of castor oil packs.

To be sure, we would not use the packs during the menstrual periods. . .
When the body has a fever it is well to apply packs.   728-2

The headaches we would relieve more with the application of the oil packs. This will aid the body.   2434-3

The following readings offer further information on the function of the castor oil packs:

The effect of these oil packs is to enliven, through the activity of the absorption through the perspiratory system, the activities in such natures and measures as to produce a greater quantity (than at present) and a superficial activity of the lymph circulation; hence setting up drainages to such measures that the poisons will be eliminated from the system...   631-4

Or there may be the use of hot castor oil packs that may assist in so dissolving the gravel in the gall duct and the gall bladder that it might be drained osteopathically, after a long series. This would require a much longer period but would be a much safer manner.   3160-1

From *every* condition that is of true epileptic nature there will be found a cold spot or area between the lacteal duct and the caecum. Over this area every other day, in the afternoon when the body rests from its physical exercise in the open, apply castor oil packs, for a period of at least *two* times every other day...We will break up the tendency for the lymph ducts, in the ducts of the lacteals and in the caecum and colon (ascending here), that tendency for contraction and for the activities that help to bring on the conditions that produce incoordination to the nerve forces of the body.   567-4

For more information, consult the CF on Castor Oil Packs or other appropriate Files such as Gall Bladder and Duct: Stones; Epilepsy; Constipation; Colitis; Cirrhosis; and Torpid Liver. See also *Edgar Cayce and the Palma Christi,* a book by Dr. William McGarey, A.R.E. Clinic, Inc.

CASTORIA (FLETCHER'S)

Castoria is a mild laxative consisting of senna in a syrup base. The readings almost always specified the use of Fletcher's Castoria, which has been in existence since the late 1800s or perhaps even earlier. This preparation was suggested in almost 150 readings, for children and adults, to gently assist sluggish excretory systems, improving the digestion in the process.

The Cayce source often expounded on the benefits Castoria would have, if properly administered. When asked about the best laxative for a one-and-a-half-year-old child, he replied: "None better than that of Castoria!" (299-3) And in another reading for a child the same age, he explained, "For the active principles, of course, are in the senna—which will work with the digestive forces, the kidneys and the activities in the liver proper. . ." (786-2)

Other readings further explained that the active properties in Castoria would be absorbed into the system, thereby sweetening the gastric flow, toning the digestion, softening the lobes of the liver, aiding the gall bladder, and cleansing the entire intestinal tract. Moreover, this cleansing would take place without causing any undue strain to the system.

The secret to obtaining these results is to take small, frequent doses. The amounts and regularity of these doses were sometimes specified and at other times left up to the individual. When specified, instructions varied somewhat with age and other factors. A reading for a nine-month-old child, for example, suggested doses of three to five drops given at fifteen- to twenty-minute intervals. For older children, the dose was about doubled, to five to ten drops or a fourth of a teaspoon every half hour. A typical adult dosage was half a teaspoon every half hour, though sometimes the intervals between doses were longer.

The Castoria was typically to be taken in this way until the alimentary canal had fully responded, resulting in one or more bowel movements. For adults, this often meant taking an entire bottle throughout the course of a day or a little longer. Resting during this time was frequently advised. Castoria dosage was often to be preceded or followed by other treatments, many of them other compatible stimulants to the eliminations.

Castoria was found particularly useful in congested or toxic systems, where rapid drainage was needed. The variety of conditions in which it was recommended included baby care, colds, colitis, liver problems, and worms.

For more information consult the appropriate CFs.

CEREALS

Of the cereals mentioned in the Cayce readings, cracked wheat and steel cut oats were perhaps the most often recommended. These cereals are higher in vitamins and minerals than the processed types.

[Take] oatmeal that is cooked a long time, not the oats cooked only a few minutes—that isn't very good for anyone. These are much better if they are of the whole grain and not rolled or so treated chemically as to cause them to cook easily.   3326-1

The use of steel cut oats was stressed in preference to rolled oats because the rolling presses out the valuable oils, whereas in the steel cut oats the oils, and hence the oil-soluble vitamins A and E are preserved.

The readings emphasized that these cereals should be cooked a long time to make them easily digestible. One method of doing this is to bring the cereal to a boil and then pour the cereal and boiling water into a widemouth thermos, which is closed and left overnight, cooking the cereal completely.

Citrus fruit juices were not to be taken at the same meal with cereals.

CHAMOMILE

Chamomile is an herb with many uses, commonly employed as a stimulant and digestive aid. It is found mentioned about twenty times in the readings for a diversity of ailments, recommended most often for stomach ulcers, psoriasis and indigestion. Often chamomile tea was to be alternated with others, such as saffron tea and elm water.

Reading 2176-1 advised that "Most, or practically all the

water that would be taken by the body should either carry those properties of elm, saffron or chamomile." The same reading gave directions for preparing the tea:

A heaping teaspoonful of the [chamomile] to six to eight ounces of water, allowed to steep until there is about four to six ounces of water—see? Then when ready to take (and this may be kept in a cool place, or on ice) put a teaspoonful of the tea (of course, strained) in a glass of water.   2176-1

Another method is to add boiling water to a pinch of chamomile in a teacup and steep for fifteen minutes before taking.

One reading comments that "Chamomile tea and saffron tea altered [alternated] from time to time...will settle the stomach and make for the releasing of the irritations." (712-1)

For more information, consult the CFs on Skin: Psoriasis, Stomach: Indigestion, and Stomach: Ulcers.

CHARCOAL TABLETS

Charcoal tablets were prescribed in about 15 readings for digestive problems and flatulence. The brand recommended was known as Kellogg's, made by Battle Creek Sanitorium. These tablets, made with willow charcoal and honey, are no longer available from any manufacturer. Other brands of charcoal tablets on the market, such as Requa's, are a possible substitute.

CHARRED OAK KEG

The charred oak keg is part of a rather unorthodox treatment recommended about 50 times in the readings, primarily in cases of tuberculosis and pleurisy. This treatment involves the placing of 100-proof apple brandy in the keg and then regularly inhaling the fumes that arise from this liquid. Charred oak kegs are used commercially in storage of aging liquors since the charcoal absorbs impurities from the liquor. This is no doubt one of the reasons that Cayce stressed keeping the brandy in the keg. Even so, the keg must be periodically rinsed with water to remove acids that have accumulated:

Before using again, "Rinse with *warm*—not hot but *warm* water, so that the accumulations from the distillation or evaporation of the properties are removed, and there is less of that influence or force which arises from the acids that come from such infusions [apple brandy]." (1548-4)

The alcohol in the brandy is an antiseptic for the lungs. According to the readings these inhalations can not only destroy tubercule tissue, but have other beneficial effects on the body as well:

The activity on this is not only for the destruction of live tubercule tissue, but it acts as an antiseptic for all irritated areas; also giving activity to cellular force of the corpuscle itself. It acts as a stimuli to the circulation, then, recharging each cell as it passes through areas so affected by the radiation of the gases from this fluid itself. 3176-1

For the properties inhaled will work with the activity of the respiratory system, as well as the properties contained therein will act upon the influences of the liver and kidneys in their ability to be purified—in the assimilating of these forces that arise from the infusion of these influences indicated.
1557-1

This will act not only as an antiseptic, but will so change the lung tissue as to bring about healing of the lung tissues, and will also increase the abilities of assimilation, and we will have improvement. 5053-1

These [inhalations] will irritate at first, but use through the nostril for the stopping of cough, as well as inhaling into the lungs. 3594-1

Do not attempt to inhale too much in the beginning, or it will be inclined to produce too much intoxication for the body.
2448-1

Keep the *keg*. This *is* as life itself. 1548-4

For more information, consult the CFs on Tuberculosis and Lungs: Pleurisy.

It is recommended that you consult a physician before using this product.

CIMEX LECTULARIUS

Cimex Lectularius is an illustration of the premise that even the most useless-seeming creatures in nature have value when put to the proper use. This product, recommended about ten times in the readings for dropsy, phlebitis and nephritis, is a homeopathic remedy made from bedbug juice.

The majority of readings suggested Cimex (which is the scientific name for bedbug) in cases of dropsy, which is a swelling of the feet, ankles and lower extremities, caused by infiltration of the tissues with diluted lymph fluid. The first reading to be quoted suggests that perhaps not everyone taking this should be told of its origin:

While the body may not be entirely well, were those changes made with the use of those properties that are compounded by the homeopathic profession for such conditions—which are more from the parasite combinations for swelling, and for conditions as related to the heart's action, and which will be a portion of the adrenalin nature for the heart's action, these would give the greater relief. . .
There is an outlined treatment for this specific character of condition. . .This would not be interpreted to those seeking it, but what they will do will be a brew of bedbug juice!   327-3

. . .we would obtain—from a good homeopathic physician— the little white pellets that are to control the lymph circulation, which is involved in such conditions.
To give what is the common name for same would not be very pleasant to the entity, but it is what is needed.   420-7

A report from [420], accompanying the above reading, comments that the treatment suggested was followed, resulting in "immediate relief."

Also would it be well for those properties as are given for such conditions, in the homeopathic applications be used, or what is *commonly* called (though not of that extraction) bedbug juice—though these are for such conditions. We will find that this given in minute quantities will reduce this condition.   5514-3

. . .that which may save these conditions in the present, is the administration by one of the homeopathic profession of that juice from the Cimex Lectularius. If called by the common name it might be offensive, but it is that which takes the place of atropine as might be used by one of the allopathic profession. If it is impossible to obtain this, then the use of atropine internally or by injections may be necessary—but use the other [Cimex] in preference.   1553-27

In a single instance Cimex Lectularius was recommended for nephritis, or inflammation of the kidneys. Cimex is perhaps most widely used in cases of phlebitis, characterized by inflammation of a vein.

[3572] was suffering from "a condition of phlebitis and a dropsical condition that extends even to the lower abdominal area." The reading continues:

Under the direction of a homeopathic physician we would add those properties of Cimex Lectularius. This should alleviate this condition. For there is some resistance here being kept in the body.   3572-1

For more information consult the CFs on Dropsy, Blood Vessels: Phlebitis, and Kidneys: Pyelitis and Nephritis.

It is recommended that you consult a physician before using this product.

CLARY WATER [5480-1]

Clary Water is a tonic that the Edgar Cayce readings suggested using in about 100 cases involving various problems associated with the assimilating and eliminating systems, including disturbances in the hepatic circulation. It was most often recommended for diabetes and hyperglycemia, and to improve the functioning of the digestion, eliminations and kidneys. One formula commonly used was given in reading 953-1, and the active ingredients are garden sage (also known as Clary Flower—hence the name Clary Water), which aids the digestion; juniper oil, which stimulates the kidneys; and ambergris, which acts on the pancreas. Additional information on these substances can be found in the readings:

. . .garden sage acts upon the liver and the pancreas in such measures and manners not to increase the gastric flow beyond that which is of a stimulating nature, and acts with the food properties taken at the time in such a way as to make for better assimilations throughout the activities of the glands and the secretions necessary for the carrying on of the gastric flow in the digestive system.

And the ambergris acts directly with the activity of the pancreas itself, making for a better association of activities between the spleen, the pancreas, and the liver; thus aiding where those pressures in the system have caused a dilatory activity through these, or increased activity of the pancreas and a slow activity of the spleen itself and to the liver for a normal flow and activity. 816-1

...ambergris acts in the human system as that necessary for the juices or the excretions from the pancreas to not turn so much sugar in the system—acting, then, in a way and manner as do those properties as are secreted by the pancreas proper *or* the pancrean fluid concentrated and reacted in the system through that of hypodermic... 953-26

Oil of juniper is "the active principle *in* gin, for the clarifying of the kidney and the hepatic circulation." (1739-1)

While Clary Water is being taken, several dietary precautions should be observed. Reading 4414-2 states, "*Do not eat meats of any character while this is being taken.*" Reading 3722-1 says to avoid sugars and proteins. Large quantities of starches and all fried foods should also be avoided, although seafood is acceptable. These foods tend to work in opposition to the Clary Water.

...as an assistant to the digestive forces in the system, those we would find in Clary Water... 3-1

Clary Water will also "tone the stomach..." (4332-1) It was also used "To produce perfect eliminations as far as possible to create within this body," (226-1) and to "make for impulses in the activity of the glandular system that would create the better balance for the body." (1422-1) For an individual suffering from progressive debilitation due to tuberculosis, one reading advised: "To assist the stomach in its digestive functions, we must use Clary Water, because it is a compound which will increase the digestive powers, and the appetite." (5707-1) This will be a "toning for the whole body, and for the digestive organ, then, the stomach will be able to take into it enough to assist the blood to build up the body, but it cannot so long as it won't digest anything." (5707-1)

In reading 1100-17 Clary Water was suggested occasionally as a substitute for Jerusalem artichokes, frequently recommended in cases of diabetes.

Formula and dosage vary somewhat from reading to reading. Once objectives have been achieved, and the blood sugar level is normal, or assimilations have been improved, then the dosage should be reduced to a level necessary to maintain the results obtained. Thereafter, the Clary Water need be taken only once daily, or whenever the need is felt. To achieve the desired results, the readings usually suggested continuing with the initial dosage prescribed until a quart had been consumed.

On Oct. 9, 1931, [5480] wrote in a letter to Gladys Davis: "In Mr. Cayce's reading he mentioned or recommended Clary Water. This we are unable to obtain in. . .Kindly give me the manufacturer's name and address as I have already started the osteopathic treatments and am anxious to make the treatment complete. Was pleased with the accuracy of the reading as regards symptoms and am following carefully all of his instructions. . ."

On Oct. 12, 1931, Edgar Cayce answered: "In reply to yours of the 9th addressed to Miss Davis, I wish to give you the formula for preparing the Clary Water.

"Put 6 ounces of the Clary Flower (or garden sage, dried) in 32 ounces of distilled water. Reduce by slow boiling, or steaming, to one-half the quantity. Strain while warm and add:

    1 ounce simple syrup,
    15 grains ambergris, dissolved in
    1 ounce of grain alcohol,
    8 ounces Gordon gin,
    1 dram Cinnamon (preferably in the stick).

"Shake solution together before dose is taken.

"You will be able to obtain the ambergris from either Lehn & Fink or Eimer & Amend. [N.Y.C.]

"I certainly hope the information will assist you to gain the health desired. Be sure to let us hear from you if we can be of any service. Also let us know how you progress. . ."

Apparently the above formula for preparing Clary Water was first given for Mr. [5676] in the fall of 1902. (See pp. 137 and 145 of *There Is a River* by Thomas Sugrue.)

Additional information about ambergris is found in dictionaries. From the current *Webster's* comes this definition: "A waxy substance found floating in tropical seas, and as a morbid secretion in the sperm whale, whence it is all believed to come. It is valued in perfumery." And in an old medical dictionary is found this information: "A biliary or intestinal concretion of the sperm-whale, *Physeter macrocephalus*. It exhales a fragrant, musky odor when warmed, and is used in adynamic fevers, chronic catarrh and nervous diseases. Dose 1-3 gr. (0.065-0.2 Gm.)." For some years now, due to restrictions against disturbing the whale, an endangered species, the ambergris is unobtainable. Ambergris is derived from whales, although ironically, a whale need not necessarily be slaughtered to obtain it.

For more information, consult the CFs on Diabetes and Stomach: Indigestion. It is recommended that you consult a physician before using this product.

COCA-COLA SYRUP

Many health food enthusiasts have reservations regarding the readings' recommendations of such a slickly advertised brand of sugar-water as Coca-Cola. Even elsewhere in the readings, soft drinks in general are found referred to as "slop." Coca-Cola's distinguishing feature lies in the manner of usage. Firstly, it is to be used as a medicine rather than a beverage, and should be taken in prescribed, limited quantities, no more than three or four times a week. The other important difference is that the Coca-Cola drinks prescribed by the Cayce source were seldom to be taken in carbonated form. The readings advised purchasing the pure syrup and then adding plain water to it in the proportion desired. Coca-Cola is an alkalizer and a diuretic, and was recommended in about six readings for kidney and bladder disorders:

To be sure, Coca-Cola is helpful to the kidneys, but if taken, use the Coca-Cola syrup in plain water—and this to the body will not be very palatable.   2332-1

Do take Coca-Cola occasionally as a drink, for the activity of the kidneys, but do not take it with carbonated water. Buy or have the syrup prepared and add plain water to this. Take about one half ounce or one ounce of the syrup and add plain water. This [is] to be taken about every other day, with or without ice. This will aid in purifying the kidney activity and bladder and will be better for the body.   5097-1

Here we find that Coca-Cola will be good, even for this baby [two years old]. This will act to purify the circulation between the kidneys and the liver. Preferably use this in plain water, however, *not* carbonated water. Have the syrup and make it with the plain water, *not* carbonated or charged water. The effect of the tannic forces will be helpful for this condition [eczema].   3109-1

For more information consult the CF on Kidneys.

COCOA BUTTER

Cocoa butter is derived from cocoa beans and was recommended about 185 times in the readings as a massage ingredient, to be used either by itself or in combination with other substances. Only readings from the major categories mentioned will be quoted here.

Baby Care:

For the developing bodies of babies and young children, cocoa butter was highly recommended as a massage, particularly along the spine. This was usually to be done once a day, after the morning or evening bath.

The parents of one child were told to daily "massage the spine well with cocoa butter; not so much as to become disturbing, but sufficient that the properties may be absorbed by the system. Also massage this down the limbs, especially the underside... This as we find should keep the body in its correct developing stages." (2289-1)

For another child of one-and-a-half years, this suggestion was given:

For the better development of the circulation through the head and through the upper portion of the body, each evening when ready for retirement—for at least a period of ten days to two weeks—we would massage with cocoa butter along the upper dorsal and cervical area. The vibrations of this with the muscular system and with the blood supply will prevent the congestions in the area, that would make for disturbances.

773-2

Frequent cocoa butter massages can in many cases be kept up for periods of several months with beneficial results. For a baby of three months, the following advice was given:

After the bath of morning, it would be well occasionally to gently massage the whole of the cerebrospinal system—one time with olive oil, the next time with cocoa butter.

These, as we find, are the better for the developments through those periods of the body's activity for the next six to eight months.

2015-4

And, for [2781]:

This will strengthen the body, strengthen all those centers from which there is the radial activity of impulses of nerve forces and of eliminations. This would be well.   2781-2

Abnormal Children:
    Many of the emotional and perceptual difficulties suffered by children originate, according to the Cayce source, through some kind of physical imbalance. Sometimes a great deal of aid can be found in daily massage, to quiet the nerves and increase circulation in certain vital areas. Cocoa butter was often recommended for this massage. Usage parallels that advised for baby care. In preference to an operation this suggestion was given for a ten-year-old boy with brain damage:

For the removal of the pressure, being part of the brain lesions. . .Massage with cocoa butter around head. . .clear to the end of the spine. This done, even once a week, will bring ease to the body.   5038-1

Breasts:
    If the readings are correct, normal breast development can be encouraged by means other than silicone injections—cocoa butter massage is simpler, much less expensive, and has no side effects. Sluggish glandular development can apparently sometimes be stimulated in such a manner with visible results, as in the following cases:

Q-2. Why have my mammary glands never developed properly, and may anything be done to cause normal bust development?
A-2. This condition is the suppression of the glandular force from the thyroid as pertaining to the mammary glands. We would massage these glands occasionally with cocoa butter— not a deep massage, but along the edge of the glands on the body that come down under the arms, you see, then about the breasts—at the base of same. This, with the glandular force purified [with Atomidine*] and the circulation set up by the correction of the deflection through the dorsal areas, will make the normal development.   2680-1

Q-3. What explanation for right breast being larger than left, and how remedy?
A-3. This is a nominal condition that exists in most individuals. If there is the desire for increasing the lesser, massage the lower portion with cocoa butter. If there is the

---

*It is recommended that you consult a physician before using this product.

33

desire to decrease the other, massage with cocoa butter adding the water from alum in same. Do this each evening. 1206-15

For more information, consult the CF on Baby Care and Children: Abnormal.

COCOA BUTTER AND QUININE OINTMENT [5188-1]

During World War II, a young staff sergeant in the U.S. Air Force requested a physical reading from Edgar Cayce. He was stationed at Henderson Airfield, Guadalcanal, the Solomons, in the southwest Pacific. One of his questions was: "Have I any trace of malaria; how can it be prevented?" Another: "Can anything be done to cause better sight in left eye?" He had also requested a life reading appointment. Edgar Cayce must have known that he would not be able to give the life reading, because this brief physical reading encompassed much that was on the mind and heart of the young man:

We have those conditions and activities which are parts of the consciousness of this entity, [5188].

Let the body keep those attitudes of constructive forces in its experience, knowing—as it enters into these activities—it is not for self but that others may know that freedom which comes with a greater knowledge of the Prince of Peace, of the Son, of the Father-God who gave the expression of self in the earth in such measures that He brought sight to the blind, the ability to restore the lame, even overcome death itself!

These keep in thy consciousness—that in Him ye live, move and have thy being, wholly. Then with every experience, every doubt, every fear (not that it is within self to doubt; yet ye may if ye trust in the shortness of thine own arms or hands, but trusting wholly in Him)—ye will come to the more perfect way, the perfect understanding, the perfect interpretation of the meaning of life.

For, life itself is the manifestation of that divine influence. Not that ye become as one gloomy, sad, but rather be joyous in the Lord, and these will not only bring greater blessings to thee in thy vision but in thy ability to meet the infections which may come from those malarial conditions from the swamp or from the mosquito. All of these ye can put aside, trusting only in the Christ.

Occasionally *do* massage along the spine with cocoa butter; that is, an ounce in which there has been put five grains of quinine, mixed thoroughly. Massage this along the spine, under the arms and in the groin. Not only will the mosquito not bite but there will be no malaria. These are not as an omen but are those influences which will keep the body in attune with the infinite.

Know that the Lord doeth all things well. Keep His law. For it is not beyond understanding if ye seek not to have thine own way, but can truly in heart, in mind and body, daily say: "Thy will, O God, be done in me and through me, daily."

We are through.   5188-1

Gladys Davis made the following notation: In answer to my inquiry, Mr. [5188] wrote on Oct. 4, 1949: "I was in the tropics for 32 months. Though I repeatedly tried to get quinine from the army medical officers, they would not let me have any. I was therefore unable to use the ointment. I did, however, follow the first suggestion 'trusting only in the Christ.' I did not contract malaria or other wounds. And I went through my tour of duty with a greater peace of mind than I had known before. If for no other reason than this, I shall be forever thankful to Edgar Cayce and the A.R.E. Sorry I could not give you a definite statement on the ointment." Mr. [5188] and his mother [3246] have remained active sponsoring members all these years (they are now life members) and have contributed generously to the furthering of the "work." Not only that, many others have found help from this formula; it can be prepared by a druggist as needed. Some have claimed it is a miraculous remedy for various topical infections, besides being a mosquito and insect repellant.

See the CF on Malaria.

COCONUT OIL SOAP

Coconut oil soap was recommended in one known reading. This individual was advised to use the Black & White creams "after a thorough cleansing with any good toilet soap, perferably that prepared with olive oil, or coconut oil rather than other characters of fats." (3051-3)

For more information, consult the CF on Skin: Complexion.

CODIRON

Codiron was a dietary supplement recommended in readings for a little over 100 individuals. Its body-building qualities were most often recommended in cases of general debilitation, poor assimilation (and elimination), anemia, toxemia and congestion.

Presumably Codiron was a combination of cod liver oil and iron. Cod liver oil is derived from the livers of certain species of fish and is regarded as useful in treating diseases of the bone, various forms of tuberculosis, and many types of general malnutrition. Iron is regarded mainly as a blood builder and its salts are used to treat anemia. Both substances are useful in themselves, and it may be that the combination is especially beneficial. However, no known substitute for the Codiron preparation presently exists.

COLDS LINIMENT [2036-6]

In about 285 readings a liniment was prescribed, consisting of equal parts melted mutton tallow (sometimes also called mutton suet), spirits of camphor and spirits of turpentine. Some variations include the addition of tincture of benzoin. This liniment was recommended primarily in cases of cold and congestion, poor circulation and kidney disorders. The readings explain that the mutton tallow penetrates and opens the pores of the skin, thus allowing the healing properties of the turpentine and camphor to be quickly absorbed.

Colds:

In cases of colds, attention to the feet and lower extremities was particularly stressed in the readings. Often the application of heat in combination with the Colds Liniment was advised. This can be done by warming the liniment prior to use, by soaking the feet prior to the application in very hot water to which mustard or pine oil may be added, by wrapping the feet afterwards in warm towels, or all of the above.

We would also rub these [substances] over the lower portion of the feet, bottoms of the feet, toast them, as it were, before the fire or before any heat that will make for the drawing of the circulation towards these portions.   304-33

It would be well that there be counterirritations more to the feet and lower limbs, than to the upper portion of the body... spirits of turpentine, spirits of camphor and mutton tallow— about equal parts, but keep them hot; and when rubbed on soles of feet and lower limbs it would be well that they be wrapped in hot towels, hot cloths or blankets.   265-8

Application to the chest and throat area was also frequently advised:

Apply about head, ears and neck an equal combination of mutton tallow, turpentine and camphor. Keep it as warm as possible without burning; until there is the draining of same—either from nasal passage, throat or ears.   2036-6

The Colds Liniment can be generally indicated whenever and wherever congestion is present in the system:

For this particular condition (that is, the congestion) we would, at least once or twice a day, massage the soles of the feet, the throat, bronchi, head and the soft tissue, or over the portions in the head of the soft tissue or antrum, and the like, with equal parts of turpentine, mutton tallow and spirits of camphor. This will tend to relax those portions of [the] system and allay the humor that is created by the excitement in the bloodstream (causing temperature) and allow the congestion from various portions of the body to be thrown more and more by the circulation into the eliminating channels. This should only be done while the congestion is apparent, or until the congestion has been entirely eliminated or relieved.   278-2

Circulation:
The Colds Liniment was variously referred to in the readings as a counterirritant and an astringent. This indicates one of its primary functions: the drawing of additional circulation to the area to which it is applied. The use of heat also increases the circulation.

At times when the lower limbs give trouble, and there is aching through the lower portion of the back, it would be well to *warm* same (although it is already warm) by the oil rubs, or by rubbing with a combination of equal parts [melted] mutton tallow, turpentine, spirits of camphor and compound tincture of benzoin. This combination rubbed into the bottoms of the feet also would be well. It will alter or change the circulation.
556-5

Also the massaging of the bottoms of the feet with that compound suggested, and rubbing from the lower limbs and knees downward with same, should aid in re-establishing better circulation.   556-6

Kidneys:
The Colds Liniment was found to be valuable in helping to

restore normal functioning to the kidneys. It was to be massaged into the base of the spine over the kidney area, and sometimes over the abdomen as well. Then heat was to be applied in the form of hot salt packs, or sometimes an electric heating pad, although "even if it is just massaged in, without the heat, it would be very beneficial." (916-2)

Reading 632-5 recommended massage with the Colds Liniment followed by heated salt packs applied on both the back and front at the same time:

...should there become distresses through the kidney area... These will *relieve* the pressure and the strain.

There will be the necessity of making for something of a counterirritant, externally, to those tendencies of the kidneys for their inflammatory conditions that arise at times; thus producing—through the activity of the bladder and the regular system as it attempts to eliminate—a preventative from these conditions becoming centralized or localized into a condition that would attempt to react or create an activity within itself.

632-6

These would make for an activity that would cause the kidneys to eliminate, and with the elimination of these cause the reduction of the temperature. . .   916-1

For more information consult the several CFs on Kidneys and the File on Colds.

COUGH SYRUP [243-29]

In reading 243-29 a cough syrup formula was given, which has since become quite popular. It was mentioned that this formula was to act "As a cough medicine, an expectorant, and for a healing through the whole system. . .It will allay the cough, *heal* those disturbing forces through the bronchi and larynx, and make for better conditions through the eliminations."

The formula contains syrup of wild cherry bark, syrup of horehound, syrup of rhubarb, elixir of wild ginger, honey and alcohol. Some of these ingredients are also given in other Cayce cough syrup formulas, and horehound and wild cherry bark particularly can be found in many cough preparations in the readings. The formula is different from the usual commercial cough syrups in that it contains a mild eliminant—rhubarb.

Other readings offer additional comments on the cough syrup ingredients:

. . .wild cherry bark is a direct activative force upon the pneumogastrics and the pulmonary system.   1012-1

Wild cherry bark is an expectorant and a purifier as combined especially with other ingredients for the blood supply.   643-1

The taking of those properties indicated for the allaying of cold and congestion—as in the cherry, the horehound—will not only aid *digestion* but stimulate the circulation for the upper portion of the head and through the bronchial area, thus giving a better flow of circulation for the throat and the gums...   808-3

The rhubarb will tone the activity of the lacteal ducts and thus aid in preventing these great strains at this time.
          543-21

. . .[wild] ginger. . .will work directly with the gastric flow in the liver's activity. . .   1019-1

Grain alcohol is a carrier for the other ingredients as well as a natural preservative, and honey, according to Cayce, aids in the assimilations. A great advantage of this formula is that it does not produce side effects and may be taken as often as once every hour until relief is obtained.

Users of this cough syrup formula have reported excellent results. In many cases it has been used with success after other cough remedies failed to bring relief.

See the CF on Colds; also the *Individual Reference File* (I.R.F.), pp. 97-98; and in Dr. Reilly's book, the section on "The Common Cold."

CRUDE OIL

Crude oil was recommended in about 30 readings as part of treatment for and prevention of baldness, dandruff and related hair and scalp problems. The following are some typical quotes from the readings for falling hair:

Q-10. Can anything be done to improve the growth of hair on my head?

A-10. This has reached those conditions, by the lack of the flow of circulation, where much of that has been destroyed from which the activities of the glands in the thyroids and the adrenals make for the stimulation to these activities. But with the corrections made [osteopathically], and with the use of such a stimulating to the scalp as crude oil with the white Vaseline and alcohol (that we have indicated through these sources), there will be stimulated a growth that will not only improve the condition but prevent further inroads of this lack of circulation in the scalp. Such a scalp treatment would be given in this way and manner:

About once each month have a *crude oil* shampoo, preferably done by self—it is messy, but it is necessary for the stimulation from the pure crude oil. Then cleanse same with the twenty percent *grain* alcohol—not wood alcohol, but *grain* alcohol—to remove the tar, the oil, and such influences, although some of the oil will have struck in sufficient to stimulate the circulation to the growth of the roots of the hair itself. Then use occasionally a little white Vaseline. The *massage* is the more important for it, you see.

Q-11. *How long should the crude oil stay on [the head] before cleansing with the alcohol solution?*

A-11. This depends, of course, upon the circumstances. For half to three quarters of an hour, if possible.   816-1

The reason *grain* alcohol is preferred to the denatured variety is given in reading 275-30: ". . .this will not *dry*—as does that which has been denatured."

A diet that works with the glands of the thyroid and especially with the sweat glands of the body would be more efficient; hence when such a scalp treatment is given there should ever be the suggestion that at least two or three meals a week should consist of seafoods; no fried or very greasy diet at all, or no fried meat at all; skins of Irish potatoes rather than the pulp. Such a diet together with an application to the scalp or to the skin will be much more efficacious in growth of hair...

Q-3. *Please give me a better and sure formula and the treatment for bald heads.*

A-3. There has never been a better than the crude oil treatment. This would be given about two or three times each month, followed with a cleansing with a twenty percent solution of grain alcohol and then massaging white Vaseline into the scalp in such a manner as to leave the whole surface of the scalp not too greasy, but as sufficient into the scalp to produce the better application of whatever may be used. But this will grow hair on *most* bald heads, unless—as we have indicated—it is of the germ nature that has destroyed the bulbs that *grow* hair. But this will prevent four-fifths of all types of disorder, and will be especially efficient with such a diet as outlined; and occasionally specific gland treatment.   636-1

Out of 22 cases of baldness quoted in the CF, eight recommended Atomidine* and other related treatments for glandular disturbance.

For treatment of dandruff, the following recommendation was given:

Use crude oil, cleansing with a twenty percent solution of *grain* alcohol. Then massage just a small portion or quantity of white Vaseline into the scalp. This will cure *any* dandruff, unless it is produced—of course—by acne or some skin disorder.   850-2

The crude oil treatment may be followed with a normal shampoo, although many readings fail to mention this. Castile or olive oil shampoo may be the best types of shampoo for this purpose, as they were frequently suggested for general use.

The use of only the crude oil that is pure and unrefined was often stressed. Confusion can result from the fact that crude oil occurs naturally in a variety of thicknesses and shades of color. Any of these may be used, presumably with equal effectiveness, so long as they are unrefined and free of additives. Some individuals prefer the honey-colored Pennsylvania grade crude oil as it has a milder odor and is easier to wash out of the hair. This variety of crude oil is paraffin-based, and some samples may appear cloudier than others due to a greater amount of paraffin. The blacker variety of crude oil is asphalt-based, and is somewhat messier.

The crude oil treatment may, if desired, be done more frequently than the readings quoted suggest. Some individuals have reported good results using it as often as several times weekly.

For more information, consult the CF on Hair: Baldness.

DANDRUFF TREATMENT [261-2]

The exact formula given here for dandruff was recommended only once in the readings, although slightly differing

*It is recommended that you consult a physician before using this product.

variations of this treatment, including the diluted grain alcohol and the Vaseline application, were mentioned many times.

Q-5. Is any special treatment recommended for dandruff, and can it be entirely cured?

A-5. If this will be used, this may entirely cure same; to water—aqua pura, that [is] preferably of *pure* water [distilled]—to four ounces of same add twenty minims [drops] of 85 percent alcohol, with that [substance by the name] of the oil of pine, two drops. This should be rubbed thoroughly into the scalp, so that there is the proper reaction from same. Then, with this [scalp area] still damp from same, massage thoroughly into the scalp [a] small quantity of white Vaseline. Then wash the head thoroughly with that of a tar soap. Do this about once each week. It will disappear.   261-2

According to the readings, both the grain alcohol and the pine oil are active against dandruff. Both are antiseptics, and both aid in increasing the superficial circulation of the scalp. The addition of Vaseline applications and the use of pine tar shampoo make a powerful combination.

D.D.D.

The product name for D.D.D. was derived from the initials of the doctor who developed the formula shortly before the turn of the century. D.D.D. was a prescription recommended about 50 times in the readings, primarily for skin irritations such as dermatitis and pruritus, and also for leg ulcers, psoriasis, eczema, hookworm, bites, hives, and poison ivy. The manufacturers suggested additional uses. D.D.D. was manufactured in solution form (regular and extra strength), cream, and soap. Readings suggesting D.D.D. lotion were referring to the liquid, and those prescribing the ointment referred to the cream. In some cases, as in the following quotation, the cream was preferred because of its gentleness to the skin, and was recommended the most often:

Apply *locally* the prescription D.D.D., and for this body, under the conditions, this in the form of the lotion would be not preferable, you see; but rather use the ointment. The ointment is not quite as severe, yet will allay the itching and irritation [of dermatitis].   1573-2

Dermatitis:

But when there is a great disturbance, use the ointment of prescription D.D.D. over those portions where there is a great excess of the scaly condition or eruptions on the body. 1702-1

In bathing the body, use a *good* antiseptic soap that would be helpful; and *do not let this come in contact with any other, or be used by any other hands, see?* This should be kept apart. Use either the D.D.D. soap as prepared for such, or the Cuticura soap; but use the D.D.D. ointment or cream as a massage into same. 849-46

Pruritus:

The Glyco-Thymoline may also be applied full strength to the various areas over the body where there is itching. If there is not sufficient strength in this, then the D.D.D. cream may be used for places of irritation outside. 337-28

Leg Ulcers:

The use of the D.D.D. solution. . .will aid in allaying the irritation—this put on with a tuft of cotton. 1541-5

As this product is currently no longer available, the best substitutes are probably Ray's Liquid and Ray's Ointment. See pertinent CFs.

DIATHERMY

Diathermy was a common form of electrotherapy used by many doctors and hospitals. It was a treatment method which used a high frequency electrical current to produce heat in the tissues and organs of the body. When carefully regulated for moderate periods of time, this heating had a number of therapeutic effects on the area of the body to which it was applied.

There were three forms of diathermy. The first was long-wave diathermy, which produced a current of moderately high frequency. This method usually used bare metal electrodes placed in direct contact with the skin. The second method, short-wave diathermy, used a high frequency current and produced heat in a large generalized area. It was usually applied through a spacing of air, glass, or rubber, but might also be applied by direct metallic contact. The newest form was microwave diathermy, in which a single beam of extremely high frequency electromagnetic energy was focused from a distance on the region to be treated. It was most effective for local heating. Both the long-wave and short-wave methods were apparently available in Cayce's day. Because the conventional high-powered form of long-wave diathermy interfered with AM radio reception, production of this type of machine was discontinued by international agreement around 1954.

The Edgar Cayce readings often referred to diathermy as "deep therapy." In 46% of the cases researched, emphasis was placed on using a current of low frequency while 20% mentioned what could be termed low power.

On July 5, 1978, Gladys Davis made the following notation: O.M. Wakefield, D.O., in Virginia Beach, Va., tells me that the old diathermy, which was replaced because of its interference with radio and TV stations, is a much improved machine now called a Medcolator. It is manufactured by Medco Products Co., Tulsa, Okla. It has taken the place of the old diathermy and sinusoidal, that is, the old short-wave machines.

DOG-ON-FOOT

This was a foot cream recommended in three known cases of athlete's foot. It contained salicylic acid, benzoic acid, and a substance called "thymic acid." The first two ingredients are also included in an athlete's foot formula mentioned in Saurs' *Manual of Skin Diseases*. Ray's Ointment and the Athlete's Foot Lotion [291-1] are possible substitutes.

ELECTRIC VIBRATOR

The electric vibrator was given as part of a variety of treatment regimens in about 375 readings. Its main function is the stimulation of circulation in sluggish areas, serving to relieve tensions and bring balance to the superficial circulation. Therefore, there are many types of cases in which it can be helpful, depending on where application is made.

The vibrator is used widely among persons following the crude oil treatment for baldness, as described in reading 4056-1. A scalp massage with the crude oil is advised, "using the electrically driven [vibrator] with the suction applicator."

Insomnia is another instance in which the vibrator can be helpful:

The use of the electrically driven vibrator should make for the relaxing sufficiently for the body to fall to sleep. Use this over the cerebrospinal system, or around the back of the head, the neck, across the shoulders, even down to the lower portion of the body, as has been indicated.   728-2

This will not only make for a stimulating of the circulation but will relax the body sufficiently to gain better recuperative forces with the rest.   313-18

Use of the electric vibrator was frequently recommended in cases involving poor eliminations. Mr. [389], suffering from headaches arising from an incoordination between the assimilating and eliminating systems of the body, was told:

These [headaches] arise as much from the digestive forces as from any other thing, and as we find with the change of the diet and the use of the vibrator as indicated, electrically driven, you see—using the cup [applicator], especially above the diaphragm area or throughout the whole...or as to produce a percussion or suction or drawing—given just before retiring— these would make for the inclinations for the body to rest better, and relieve the headaches.   389-9

Imbalances in the eliminating functions can be temporarily relieved without strain on the system through use of the vibrator:

In the evenings also before retiring, the use of the electrically driven vibrator along the whole cerebrospinal system will be found to be helpful; for this will enable all centers along the cerebrospinal system to receive a greater impulse from their activity, enabling all organs to be stimulated without the excess of one's functioning so much under the strain of the tautness of another...

The vibrations given in the electrically driven vibrator are to stimulate those centers (with this enlivening of the organs of the body in the digestive and eliminating system) from the nerve plexus along the cerebrospinal system, so that their activity [may] produce nearer a normal impulse than is exercised by taking large quantities of cathartics—that will relieve the pressures for the moment, but not the causes.

265-6

For individuals suffering from spinal lesions—that is, structural or functional alterations due to injury—the vibrator was sometimes recommended as an aid to restoring normal alignment:

...the vibration will act as the stimulation to those portions along the system, see, from the middle of the spine to the base of the brain—*deep!* It should be given not with the sponge but with the hard applicator, see, and go deep—along each side of the cerebrospinal system. This will make for a muscular relaxation and contraction that will make for the *adjustments* necessary... 306-1

The vibrator was recommended most frequently in cases of subluxations of the spine—incomplete dislocations or sprains:

To correct the system we only need to produce the vibration necessary to make the equalization of the nerve pressure through muscular forces over the system, and we will correct or bring the normal forces to this body... 4101-1

And, for incoordination of nervous systems:

Also we would find that the electrically driven vibrator would be excellent for quieting the nerve forces of the body... 369-10

The vibrator can help "conditions throughout the system [to] be relieved from the tension under which the nerve forces are operating or working, and will be most beneficial." (140-35)

In cases of general debilitation caused by illness or age, use of the vibrator was often suggested:

To quiet the body at times we would use the sponge applicator of the electrically driven vibrator...This as we find will relax the body, and—with the oil rub and the Radio-Active Appliance* for stimulating equalized circulation—we will materially aid and strengthen the body. 326-12

When applied in combination with the use of oils in massage, the vibrator can be especially effective in promoting normal circulation. In reading 2452-2 a *deep* massage with peanut oil along the spine is advised:

Then, following such a massage, apply the electrically

*It is recommended that you consult a physician before using this product.

driven vibrator; using the cup applicator to *draw* the circulation to those areas in which the application is made, so that the absorbing of the oil has a better distribution through the general muscular as well as regular circulation. Do not just lightly pass the cup applicator over the body, but use it in such a manner as to draw the circulation to the areas. This, we find, will materially aid if applied in this way and manner.

And, as with all Cayce treatments, the following advice applies generally:

When this is given, do not take it or have it given just as something to be gotten through with, but to be an exercise that will make for a helpfulness and an aid to creating the proper balance. 1196-9

The electric vibrator attachments mentioned in the readings correspond to the attachment names of present-day vibrators as follows:

Cayce's Name	Present-Day
Suction	Facial
Sponge	Facial
Hard	Body
Cup	General

ELIMINATIONS STIMULANT [4288-1]

This herbal tonic was recommended in a reading for a woman with high blood pressure. Cayce attributed this condition to poor eliminations, which had created an excess of toxins in the blood, and thus increased the blood pressure. Toxins in the digestive tract were reflexly affecting the liver and kidneys, causing trouble in the extremities and other areas.

The purpose of the tonic was to stimulate the eliminations and normalize the blood pressure. As the reading put it, "This is to produce elimination through the kidneys and carry functioning through the system to relieve through the dross, see." This would "give full balance to the system and make the body efficient in its physical force..." (4288-1)

This formula contains sarsaparilla root, wild cherry bark, burdock root, mandrake root, buchu leaves, grain alcohol, and balsam of tolu. Similar formulas were recommended many times in the readings.

See the CFs on Hypertension and Toxemia.

ELIXIR OF LACTATED PEPSIN

Elixir of lactated pepsin contains a digestive enzyme extracted from the stomachs of animals, such as calves, sheep or hogs. It is normally present in sufficient amounts in the human stomach, but if depleted may be taken in the form of supplements as a digestive aid.

Pepsin was recommended primarily for the digestion and assimilations, and also in cases of incoordination between assimilations and eliminations, acidity, toxemia and colitis. It was often given as a tonic ingredient in combination with various herbs, such as in the Ginseng Tonics and Formula from [636-1]. When recommended by itself, dosage given varied from three to ten drops in a glass of water taken before, after or during meals. This may be taken from one to three times a day, as needed. On the reaction of pepsin with the system, the readings offer the following comments:

...it is the reaction from this small quantity that is needed—with the activity of the hypogastric...   2474-1

...there needs to be more of those [properties taken] that will produce the tendencies for alkalinity—but more of those as may be had in the form of the essence of pepsin, or the compound known as elixir of lactated pepsin. This reaction may be had, of course, much from the use of certain vegetables; but if the body finds that these are not supplying that necessary—but that there is a tendency for the continuation of this folding up or rolling up as it were of foods in the stomach, a little of the elixir of lactated pepsin in water will be found to be helpful.   1299-1

Elixir of lactated pepsin was frequently recommended in combination with Milk of Bismuth:

The effect of same is to make for a relaxation through the pylorus, and the emptying of the stomach itself. The pepsin is to act with the lacteals to produce more of the alkalin reaction, while the Bismuth becomes an absorbent and prevents the toxic forces from giving irritation to the mucous membranes of those portions of the body through which these distresses pass; or the duodenum, and the activity of the juices from the pancreas, the activity of the gall ducts in their secretions for the preparation of foods for proper assimilation, will be stimulated.   1100-6

. . .it will be found that there will be the absorption of the poisons by the taking of the small quantity of the Milk of Bismuth (not more than a quarter teaspoonful) with the six to eight to nine drops of the elixir of lactated pepsin in half a glass of water once a day. . .

This will insure digestion, this will add to the digestive flow of the stomach itself.   667-8

For more information consult the CF on Stomach: Indigestion.

ELLIOTT TREATMENT

The Elliott Treatment was a technique intended to produce a high localized temperature through the use of water. In Cayce's day it was used medically in certain pelvic inflammatory diseases and in rectal and prostatic conditions. The readings recommended its use in a number of conditions, including sixteen cases of prostatic disorders (mostly prostatitis), six cases of nasal congestion, three cases of hemorrhoids, and one case each of oophoritis and venereal disease.

The Elliott machine consisted of a water-heating container, a motor-driven pump, and gauges and valves for the control of temperature and pressure. Vaginal and rectal applicators made of rubber were placed in these body orifices after enemas or colonics had been given to cleanse the intestinal tract. Then the introduction of water would produce a mechanical distention of up to three or four pounds of pressure, or whatever was comfortable for the patient. The temperature would begin at slightly above body heat and rise to 103° or 135°F. Treatments usually lasted half an hour and were given three times weekly.

On Feb. 22, 1945, Gladys Davis received a note from Henry George, III, D.O., Wilmington, Del., answering her question from members about obtaining the "hard-to-get" Elliott Treatment: "They are effective in certain pelvic inflammatory diseases, rectal and prostatic conditions. Because of convenience most doctors probably prefer shortwave diathermy."

See also the section on "Diathermy."

ELM WATER

Elm water received about 125 recommendations in the Cayce files, primarily in cases of poor assimilations, psoriasis and

49

stomach ulcers. It is indicated as an aid to proper digestion, as well as for such instances as those listed above in which poor digestion is a closely associated factor.

Well that occasionally those properties in the elm...be given as an easing for the conditions in the stomach proper.

2190-1

In many cases the Cayce source found that either elm or saffron water, or sometimes both, would be satisfactory and bring about similar results:

There should be no water taken unless carrying *elm bark* or *yellow saffron* tea. While these may be in small quantities, the effect of these upon the gastric flow throughout the stomach, throughout the activity of the organs of the system, will so stimulate the walls of the organs themselves as to bring *healing* to those portions that are distressed.   745-1

If the elm water causes belching, then dosage should be reduced or saffron substituted:

If this is belched, then reduce the quantity but keep on taking.   261-22

Should this become offensive, in that it produces belching from non-activity through the system, discontinue and take yellow saffron water, or tea, see?   356-1

Another reading explains why this reaction might occur:

Do not make the elm water until it is ready or just before it is ready to be drunk, for this is *easy* to become rancid. . . 348-6

Elm water is prepared by placing a pinch of the powdered slippery elm bark in a glass of cool (not ice-cold) water and letting this stand for about three minutes before taking. This may be taken once a day or, in severe cases, as often as a drink of water is desired, until conditions have been corrected.

For more information consult the CFs on Skin: Psoriasis and Stomach: Ulcers.

ENO SALTS

In the approximately 170 readings recommending Eno salts, the Cayce source sometimes specified the variety containing fruit salts (citric acid). This variety is no longer available in the United States, although it can still be found in England. However, the regular variety is still available.

EYE TONIC [3810-1]

The readings recommended herbal tonics for many and various disorders. Eye problems were no exception, although tonics were recommended only for eye problems in which poor digestion and eliminations were associated factors. The formula in reading 3810-1 was given for a 60-year-old woman suffering from toxemia who had been blind for over a year. The reading stated that to restore the sight it was first necessary to eliminate the poisons producing this condition and re-establish physical equilibrium. The reading asserted that once the correct vibrations were created in the body, the eyesight could become even stronger than was usual for those of her age.

The tonic formula contains the following herbs: sarsaparilla, yellow dock, burdock, black haw, prickly ash bark, elder flowers and tolu balsam.

While this formula was being taken, [3810] was advised to have sweat baths which would help distribute the medicinal properties throughout the body. Use of an electric vibrator to stimulate the system as well as dietary measures (plenty of green vegetables) were also suggested. This treatment, the readings claimed, would restore the sight to normal in nine weeks, implying that the formula, if taken on a daily basis, would need to be remade several times in order to provide sufficient dosage. Reports accompanying a series of readings for [3810] indicated that her condition did improve.

See the CFs on Blindness and Toxemia.

FOOT FORMULA [555-5]

A man who had a foot infection resulting from an injury was told:

In the lower portions of the extremities, where there has been the injury in the foot or the toe, these do not show infection but a stiffness.

From the hips down, rubbing on either one of the limbs or both; not over the portions that have shown injury but in the feet and in the ankle, limb and hip, a small portion of the following compound massaged into same will be most beneficial:

To 4 ounces of Russian White Oil, add:

Witch hazel .... 2 ounces
Rub alcohol .... 1 ounce
   (not wood, but *rub* alcohol compound)
Oil of sassafras .... 3 to 5 minims

Shake this together. Only use a small portion of same at the time. Begin with the hips and rub down.

This would be good for anyone that stands on the feet much, or whose feet pain, or ankle or knees or tendons.   555-5

This can be made up at home and kept on hand for use when needed.

FORMULA FROM [636-1]

This is the only formula of its kind in the Cayce readings. It was originally recommended as an aid to restoring natural color to gray hair.

The Formula from [636] is an unusual combination of herbs and other substances high in essential vitamins and minerals.

For those taking this formula specifically to restore natural color to gray hair, the use of crude oil externally to stimulate the circulation in the scalp is also suggested. Note the reference to crude oil in the underlined portion of the quotation that follows (author's italics):

Q-4. Please give me a formula for a medicine to be taken internally to restore natural color to hair.

A-4. This would necessarily be put up under the direction of a pharmacist, unless it was formed into an organization for the manufacture of same, which would be a combination in these proportions, whether making two ounces or four hundred gallons.

To four ounces of simple syrup, add:

Lactated pepsin .... 1 ounce
Black snake root extract .... ¼ ounce
Essence of wild ginseng .... ¼ ounce
Atomidine* .... 40 minims
Extract of liver (preserved in alcohol, of course, or
Armour's Liver Extract) .... ½ ounce
Grain alcohol .... ¼ ounce

The dosage of this would be half a teaspoonful three times each day, just after meals, for periods of ten days with five-day

---

*It is recommended that you consult a physician before using this product.

rest periods. This taken in such a manner over a period of several months will be effective to glands, to those secretions that will not only make a digestion that will be much improved in health but—*with any good scalp treatment, especially such as we have indicated* [crude oil]—it'll turn graying hairs back to normal; or where it has been streaked even by various forms of dyes, its *growth* will come normal. . .

To turn again to why such a formula as given would affect the body-functionings, as to change the outward activity of the functioning of glands in a body:

The syrup, surely, is the carrier.

The pepsin is active such that the ingredients given may be effective upon the basic influences within the body that would produce in the varied offices of the body those proper functionings to stimulate in the proper porportions the activities of the cuticle and the epidermis.

So the basis of not only the complexions of body would be changed as to be more healthful and thus in an activative force to beautifying of that which is to man his crown of strength and to woman her head of beauty, for to man hair in the head is as strength—to woman is as beauty.

Then the essence of the black snake root is an active principle with the lacteal ducts that make for secretions in the system that stimulate a capillary circulation; aided in same and purified through the wild ginseng essence, that is— according to the ancients—the basis of the stimulation of life in its very essence in the body of man.

The Atomidine*—that is activative in the glands, especially the thyroid, the adrenal and all the ductless activities through the atomic forces in iodine, the one basic force with potash— makes for a balance throughout the functionings of the body itself.

While the extract of liver with the preservatives, in the activities with the other portions of the body, become beautifiers. Hence, proportioned as indicated, are activative with a body—healthy; the nails, the cuticle, the epidermis, and the adorning of the beauty of the body—*beautiful!*   636-1

See the CFs on Hair; and Rejuvenation and Longevity.

GEMS AND MINERALS

Many varieties of gems and stones were found to be helpful influences in both mental and spiritual respects. A few seem to

---

*It is recommended that you consult a physician before using this product.

have had a beneficial influence on the physical bodies for whom they were recommended.

Carbon Steel:

Do not take this as being a something of superstition, or as something which would be a good luck charm, but if the entity will wear about its person, or in its pocket, a metal that is carbon steel—preferably in the groin pocket—it will prevent, it will ionize the body—from its very vibrations—to resist cold, congestion, and those inclinations for disturbance with the mucous membranes of the throat and nasal passages. 1842-1

Lapis Lazuli:

Symbols and such activities have always meant something to the entity. Hence certain characters of adornments would be well about the entity. Keep something blue, and especially the color and emanations of the lapis lazuli [about the body]; not the slick or polished nature, but of that nature that the emanations from same may give life and vitality.   2132-1

As to stones, have near to self, wear preferably upon the body, about the neck, the lapis lazuli; this preferably encased in crystal. It will be not merely as an ornament but as strength from the emanation which will be gained by the body always from same. For the stone is itself an emanation of vibrations of the elements that give vitality, virility, strength, and that of assurance in self.   1981-1

The lapis lazuli, worn close to the body would be well for the general health of the body. . .   3416-1

See the A.R.E. Press book on *Gems and Stones* for more information.

GINSENG

Wild ginseng was recommended in about 35 readings. It is an herb that was never suggested by itself, but always in combination with other herbs, such as in Formula from [636-1]* the Ginseng Tonic [2085-1]*, and Ginseng Tonic [5057-1].* *Wild* ginseng was always emphasized, as opposed to the more plentiful, cultivated variety.

---

*It is recommended that you consult a physician before using this product.

54

Ginseng has historically been valued in Oriental countries, especially China, where it is used as a cure-all for ailments ranging from sex problems to the common cold. In ancient times Chinese emperors purchased ginseng for its weight in gold, or exacted the roots as tribute from Korea.

The readings offer the following comments on the function of ginseng:

...wild ginseng...an essence of the flow of the vitality *within* the system itself. It is an *electrifying* of the vital forces themselves.   404-4

. . .increasing their [glands'] stability through the life principle as we have in wild ginseng. . .   839-1

. . .wild ginseng will act directly with these combinations [wild cherry bark, sarsaparilla root, etc.] to the activities of the glands of the system; the genitive glands, the lacteal ducts, the lachrymal ducts, the adrenals, the thyroid, all will—with these combinations—make for an activity that is purifying and body-building.   643-1

It is recommended that you consult a physician before using this product.

GINSENG TONIC [2085-1]

The formula for colitis given in reading 2085-1 has been found to be typical of the many cases in which such a tonic was recommended.

Colitis is a form of chronic diarrhea caused, in part, by inflammation of the intestinal walls, improper assimilation of foods, and toxins in the lymphatics. The tonic is directed at helping to reduce the glandular disturbance and restore a proper balance between the assimilations and eliminations:

This compound taken internally as a stimulant to the activities through the alimentary canal, with the osteopathic corrections given, will gradually make for not only the correcting of the condition but the eliminating of the causes of same; and thus bring about a near normal or equal balance in the functioning of the organs, as well as the glandular forces, and clearing gradually the disturbance wherein the activities through the whole of the alimentary canal may be eliminated and eradicated entirely from the system.   2085-1

The ingredients contained in this formula are wild ginger, wild ginseng, lactated pepsin and stillingia, and all receive frequent references in the readings.

Elixir of lactated pepsin was included in about 15 additional formulas for colitis and was also recommended in about 45 readings as an aid in digestion. In reading 556-4 pepsin is mentioned as a stimulant to the lacteal duct area, which is closely associated with the assimilatory process.

Stimulation from the wild ginseng is to the gastric flow but acts primarily upon the glands of the gastric flow for an activity to the thyroid, to the ducts and glands within the liver area itself...　　　　　　　**1019-1**

In those of the [wild] ginger and ginseng, act directly with the organs as are affected by the gland production in system.
1278-1

Stillingia...in this combination makes for an activity to the kidneys for purifying or cleansing same, thus building or purifying the blood supply and adding to the gastric flow.
1019-1

Of a similar formula containing wild ginseng, wild ginger, elixir of lactated pepsin, distilled water and alcohol, recommended to improve the eliminations, one reading stated:

...we will find we will rid the system of this tendency for the lymph—in its circulation through the alimentary canal—to be supplied and to allay those tendencies for this condition through [the] stomach and intestinal tract to upset the lymph flow in neck and head, and clear the throat.　　　**2834-2**

For more information, consult the CF on Intestines: Colitis. It is recommended that you consult a physician before using this product.

GINSENG TONIC [5057-1]

On Oct. 18, 1952, Gladys Davis made the following notation: D.H. Fogel (M.D., heart specialist), after studying several other cases from the Edgar Cayce files on colitis, including 5237-1, 5215-1, 340-23, 5178-1, 5000-2, and 5280-1, told me that the ginseng formula should be made available to A.R.E. members for this dread disease of chronic ulcerative colitis. Dr. Fogel's comment: "There is no known cure for it. Edgar Cayce says intestinal flu causes this."

Dr. Fogel then proceeded to write out the 5057-1 formula for *Chronic Ulcerative Colitis,* modified only as to directions for usage with additional regimen, as follows:

Make a fusion of wild ginseng.

Preparation: (1) Add 5 drachms of wild ginseng to a pint of distilled water. Let it come to a boil and boil until there is only ½ pint left, after straining same.

(2) Then make a fusion of this: Use 2 drachms of wild ginger in 4 ounces of distilled water. Let this come to a boil and boil until there is only 2 ounces left, after straining.

(3) Add (1) and (2) together, and add to them 4 ounces of lactated pepsin and 1 ounce of grain alcohol.

Directions: (1) One teaspoon after breakfast and at bedtime for 10 days, and leave off for 5 days, and repeat cycle until medicine is gone.

(2) Massage spine with peanut oil at least 3 times weekly.

Mrs. [5057], a 50-year-old woman who obtained her first reading on May 6, 1944, had many other serious ailments besides ulcerative colitis. Although she did not report a cure from attempting to follow the many things suggested for her, the above prescription, which Dr. Fogel extracted from that reading, has been tried and found helpful by many people.

See CF on Colitis: Ulcerative, which has several pages of supplements carrying reports from grateful A.R.E. members who, in cooperation with their physicians, used the 5057-1 Ginseng Tonic.

It is recommended that you consult a physician before using this product.

GLYCO-THYMOLINE

According to its manufacturer, Glyco-Thymoline is primarily a treatment for mucosity to be used as a spray or gargle for nasal and throat passages. In addition it is indicated—diluted with water in some cases—for smoker's cough, teeth or sore gums, false teeth or partial dentures, halitosis, superficial cuts, allergies, diaper rash, feminine hygiene, poison ivy, hives, insect bites, and sunburn. The manufacturers report that the formula has not changed since Cayce's day.

In the readings Glyco-Thymoline is referred to approximately 810 times. Many usages suggested coincide closely with label recommendations. Other readings offer several new ways it can be used.

Intestinal Antiseptic:
According to the readings, when the system is overacid, cold and congestion can easily develop. Glyco-Thymoline was sometimes recommended to restore the normal acid-alkaline balance:

Use an alkalizer for the alimentary canal. . .each day take three to four drops of Glyco-Thymoline internally in a little water. Take this for sufficient period until the *odor* [of Glyco-Thymoline] may be detected from the stool. This will purify the whole of the alimentary canal and create an alkaline reaction *through* the lower portion of the alimentary canal.   1807-3

At times there will be a cough and spittle, but in such periods take internally about two or three times a day, three drops of Glyco-Thymoline in a glass of water, as an intestinal antiseptic, as well as an absorbent of the destructive or detrimental forces coming from the cough.   5097-1

[Take]. . .three drops of Glyco-Thymoline in water before retiring at night. . .The Glyco-Thymoline acts as an intestinal antiseptic of an alkaline nature. . .   3104-1

Eyes:
Glyco-Thymoline was sometimes recommended as an application for tired or irritated eyes:

Q-1. What should be done to relieve my eyes?
A-1. Bathe them with a weak Glyco-Thymoline solution. Use an eye cup, and two parts of distilled water (preferably) to one part of the Glyco-Thymoline. This irritation is a part of the kidney disturbance that has come from the upsetting in the digestive forces.   3050-2

Packs:
Application of packs was recommended for a variety of conditions, some of these also involving the use of heat:

. . .there should be a systematic series of osteopathic adjustments. However, each time before these adjustments are made—which should be twice a week—we would relax the area to be adjusted by applying heavy packs of Glyco-

Thymoline. Use three or four thicknesses of cotton cloth saturated with warm Glyco-Thymoline and apply for at least an hour to an hour and a half, the day before the adjustments are to be made. Let these packs extend over the lumbar area and all of the sacral area, even to the end of the spine. Apply heat over this, not too much but sufficient to cause these properties not only to relax the body but to be absorbed into those areas. Thus the osteopathic corrections, when administered the next day, will relieve these tensions and make for those tendencies towards a better coordination and a better alkalinity in the eliminations. Thus the activity to the kidneys will be aided, also of the bladder and organs of [the] pelvis, as well as the activity for the whole body.   3157-1

For sinus congestion, application of a clean cloth soaked in warm Glyco-Thymoline and applied over the area can sometimes aid in rapid relief.

Colonics:
A colonic is an irrigation of the colon often given as a portion of treatment in various cases involving poor eliminations. The readings often recommended that Glyco-Thymoline be added to the final quantity of water used:

. . .have a good hydrotherapist give a thorough but gentle colon cleansing—this possibly a week or two weeks apart. In the first waters, use salt and soda, in the proportions of a heaping teaspoonful of table salt and a level teaspoonful of baking soda [both] dissolved thoroughly to each half gallon of water. In the last water use Glyco-Thymoline as an intestinal antiseptic to purify the system, in the proportions of a tablespoonful to the quart of water.   1745-4

When taking Glyco-Thymoline internally, it should be kept in mind that it is poisonous when taken in large quantities, and no more than a few drops daily should be taken.
For more information, consult the CF on Glyco-Thymoline.

GOLD CHLORIDE

Gold chloride is a solution of gold dissolved in distilled water, and is perhaps best known for its use in conjunction with the Radio-Active Appliance* and the Wet Cell Appliance.*
Many readings state or imply that it is best to add gold

*It is recommended that you consult a physician before using this product.

chloride to the system vibratorially by means of the Appliance, rather than by injection or ingestion. However, there are also about 190 readings recommending small amounts of gold chloride taken internally in combination with bromide of soda or bicarbonate of soda. Of the readings studied, about one-third recommended bicarbonate of soda, and two-thirds bromide of soda.*

The gold and soda solutions were recommended most frequently in cases of arthritis. Reading 319-1 gives a typical dosage:

When beginning to take, take one drop of the chloride of gold [1 grain/oz.] (this in half a glass of water) solution and two drops of the soda solution [usually 2 grains/oz.]. See? The next day take two drops of the gold solution and four drops of the soda solution. Increase in this manner until five days have passed.

Frequently, use of this solution was to precede a Violet Ray* (high frequency machine, bulb applicator) treatment. One reading stated that this treatment combination would aid in "Assisting the eliminations, aiding the system to function through the glands—where assimilation has been hindered, that causes tautness in the centers about nerve ends, where they join in the joints or sinews of the body." (120-2)

Some extremely interesting comments on the use of gold in cases of alcoholism were made in reading 606-1. One drop of gold solution and two drops of bromide of soda were to be taken in half a glass of water twice daily, each day increasing the dosage by one drop and two drops respectively for five days. Then:

Rest two days and then begin all over again with the one and two drops, and so on as given. . .

Q-3. Should any alcoholic stimulant be taken? If so, in what form? Beer, wine or hard liquor?

A-3. Naturally, there will be the desire. It should be gradually weakened and weakened; and four or five days— well, he won't want it—without vomiting up his shoe soles! Whether it's hard liquor or what! Alcohol won't work with gold! This is the gold treatment, but it builds the resistance.

Q-4. In alcoholic cases, can a general outline of treatment be given?

A-4. No. Each individual has its own individual problems.

*It is recommended that you consult a physician before using this product.

Not *all* are *physical.* Hence there are those that are of the sympathetic nature, or where there has been the possession by the very activity of same; but gold will destroy desire in any of them!   606-1

Treatment with gold and soda was often indicated in cases of glandular and nervous incoordination. In the following reading it was stated that gold and bicarbonate of soda "will bring about the necessary vibration for the correction in elimination of the conditions as are loosened, as it were, and allow the glands in the torso of the body to be rejuvenated... Keep these [gold and soda solutions] separate, until they are to be taken in the system." (359-1)

The action in the physical in these conditions are as these: In the mechanical or medicinal forces in [the] system [this] is to create in the nerve plasm, as gives incentive from [the] center of the nerve forces, that creative [force] that overcomes the suppression as was manifested in [the] system in times back.   4581-1

In discussing cases of insanity, the Cayce source sometimes mentioned the gold and soda, and in one reading called it the "*Gold* cure." (736-1)

In many readings recommending gold, Atomidine* was also mentioned, probably because it also affects the glands. It is important to remember that Atomidine and gold should never be taken at the same time, but may be alternated in cycles if desired.

For more information, consult the CFs on Arthritis; Alcoholism; and Rejuvenation and Longevity.

It is recommended that you consult a physician before using this product.

GRAIN ALCOHOL (20% SOLUTION)

Twenty percent grain alcohol was mentioned five times in the Cayce readings as a portion of treatment outlined for hair and scalp problems, such as baldness, falling hair, graying hair and dandruff. In three other similar cases, grain alcohol was recommended in either weaker solutions, or in unspecified proportions.

A 20% solution contains one part 190 proof (95%) pure grain

---

*It is recommended that you consult a physician before using this product.

alcohol to four parts distilled water. The readings specified that only *grain* alcohol be used; never denatured (rubbing) alcohol or wood alcohol. This solution is most often used in cases of baldness and falling hair, in conjunction with a crude oil scalp massage, as in the following reading:

The diets affect this [falling hair] principally, though those portions where this [loss of hair] is indicated would be stimulated by a massage—which may be had with properties that aid the scalp circulation; such as a small quantity of the crude oil. Rub this into the scalp once or twice a month; this should be sufficient to renew the cells that produce this—if there is the stimulation through the gastric flow in the digestive forces and the stimulation through the general distribution of the circulatory forces of the body.

Each time after the crude oil massage, when the oil is rubbed in, cleanse same with a 20% solution of alcohol—water added; grain alcohol, not those that are cut. This should be sufficient to make for a growth that is most helpful, and prevent the falling out.   480-23

Sometimes white Vaseline was also given as part of the baldness treatment:

Use as a massage the crude oil, cleansing same with a 20% solution of *grain* alcohol; not denatured or wood alcohol, but *grain* alcohol; and massage into the scalp small quantities of the white Vaseline. These will stimulate growth.   826-1

The crude oil/20% grain alcohol/white Vaseline combination can also apparently be helpful in some cases of dandruff:

Use crude oil, cleansing with a 20% solution of *grain* alcohol. Then massage a small portion or quantity of white Vaseline into the scalp. This will cure *any* dandruff, unless it is produced—of course—by acne or some skin disorder.   850-2

In two cases of falling hair, grain alcohol solutions were recommended in conjunction primarily with the white Vaseline:

Upon the scalp use such as Listerine as a wash. Then use an oil, such as the...white Vaseline; and cleanse same with a very *weak* solution of grain alcohol. This tends to make for a stimulating of the scalp circulation and to close the ends of the hairs themselves; as do the others tend to stimulate the activity to the scalp circulation.   337-24

Do this in the exterior portions of the circulation and capillaries. Use pure white Vaseline...Rub well into the parts affected. Then cleanse with a 20% solution pure grain alcohol massaged into [the] scalp of portion of body so showing this condition.   270-1

For more information, consult the CF on Hair: Baldness.

GROVE'S CHILL TONIC

This remedy, labeled as Grove's Tasteless Chill Tonic, appeared around 1900 as a remedy for malaria, chills and fever. E.W. Grove was a Tennessee pharmacist who later developed a whole line of health remedies in Chicago, the most famous of which was the Chill Tonic. Profits from this and another remedy were used to build the Grove Park Inn, which is still functioning in Asheville, North Carolina, and is listed on the National Register of Historic Places.

The main ingredient of Grove's Chill Tonic was cinchona or "fever bark," which the readings recommended as a natural source of quinine. The tonic also contained iron and lemon flavoring in a syrup base. This preparation was given about 25 times, primarily in cases of malaria, and also in other disorders, such as poor elimination and streptococcus infection. In one recommendation, the Cayce source wryly commented, "It is not very tasteless, but that's the name it is called." (2548-1) A possible substitute is one of the numerous herbal tonics in the readings which contain cinchona or calisaya as an ingredient.

HEADACHE FORMULA [263-16]

This formula was given in a reading for a person suffering from severe headaches. While additional measures were being taken to counteract the causes, a combination of equal parts of camphor and tincture of lobelia was to be applied to the temples to alleviate the pain. For best results, the user was to rest, with the eyes covered with cold cloths during application.

For more information consult the CF on Headache.

HERB TONIC [2790-1]

The husband of [2790] requested this physical reading saying that his wife was suffering from extreme nervousness and gastralgia. The herbs recommended were wild cherry bark, yellow root (also known as Golden Seal), red root, prickly ash bark, elder flowers, and balm of Gilead.

The effect of this on the system is to give the stimulation to the organs and to the eliminating forces in the system, as in this:

The active principle from the wild cherry bark, with the other ingredients, is a stimulation to the lungs, throat and bronchials, and those organs above the diaphragm.

The yellow root is for the pneumogastric forces, and gastric juices of the pyloric end of the stomach itself.

The red root is a stimulus for the secretions from the pancrean forces and the spleen, in its functioning from the blood cell force as destroyed there.

The prickly ash bark is for the blood supply, as acted upon in the emunctory forces of the liver itself, proper.

The elder flower is [for] the functioning of the organs of the pelvis with the action of the kidneys; with the stimulation from the alcohol and balm of Gilead in these organs. 2790-1

This tonic, as a whole, should act as "stimulation to the body to give the correct vibration through the system."

See the CF on Stomach: Indigestion and Gastritis. This product is no longer available.

It is recommended that you consult a physician before using this product.

HERBAL SPRING TONIC [5450-3]

On a spring day in March, 1930, a formula was given for an herbal tonic for general use. Given in reading 5450-3, the statement was made that "this would be good for everyone [who needs it] as a spring tonic." It is the *only* herbal tonic in the readings that is generally recommended, and—at least for the individual concerned—"will assist in clarifying the whole system."

The individual for whom the Herbal Spring Tonic was suggested was suffering from acne, boils and other skin eruptions, which the reading found to be internally caused. This formula contains three of the herbs most frequently prescribed in the readings: sarsaparilla root, wild cherry bark, and yellow duck root, along with dogwood bark, dogfennel, prickly ash bark, balsam of tolu, sassafras oil and tincture of capsici. Explanations of how these herbs act on the body were given in other readings:

The active principle from the wild cherry bark with the other ingredients is a stimulation to the lungs, throat and bronchials, and those organs above the diaphragm.   2790-1

The first ingredient, the wild cherry bark, is a direct activative force upon the pneumogastrics and the pulmonary system.
The sarsaparilla works with the gastric juices of the stomach, and the eliminations in the peristaltic movement through the intestinal tract.   1012-1

The yellow dock root is an emit and blood purifier, an active principle with the secretions of the liver.   643-1

The prickly ash bark acts directly with the activative forces in the liver itself, in the gall duct, and as a stimulant to the pancreas and spleen's activity.   1012-1

Sarsaparilla, wild cherry bark and yellow dock root are herbs that are frequently combined in Cayce formulas. They are tonic ingredients in about 80 different readings, dealing primarily with poor eliminations, and incoordinations between the assimilating and eliminating functions. The following reading, which prescribed a tonic containing these ingredients, also described how it should react within the system:

. . .prepare a compound to be taken internally to work with the blood supply, and to create an activity with the glands and the assimilating system as to alleviate the conditions; so that . . .the eliminations and assimilations and activity of [the] glands—through this compound of properties—may aid in creating the *correct* balance for the body.   643-1

HIGH ENEMAS AND COLONICS

Various methods of cleansing the colon were included as a portion of therapy in a large number of readings. Colonics and enemas were the means most frequently advised, not so much as curative measures but to help increase the effectiveness of other treatments applied, both in cases of illness and for general upkeep of physical health and balance. The following readings comment on the function of colonic irrigations, how frequently they should be given, and on the advisability of adding certain substances to the water used:

Q-7. How often should I take colonics?

A-7. This depends on how often they are needed. These are things that are used as aids. They are seldom curatives, unless there are those measures taken to aid in correcting the cause of the disturbance. When there is lack of the eliminations through [the] alimentary canal, then to cleanse the colon have the irrigation. Whether this is necessary once a week, twice a week, once in six weeks or once in six months, depends upon the manner in which the body treats itself. But these are well to be used when needed. If they are given body-temperature with the water used, and with the cleansing solutions in same, the salt and soda in proportions indicated, and the Glyco [-Thymoline] as the purifier—or the like—these will not be weakening but will help. But too often given, too cold or too hot a water, they will be disturbing.   303-34

After [303] was given "a colonic this morning and collapsed in [the] doctor's office," the Cayce source made the following comment in answer to this question:

Q-1. Should another colonic be taken after this period of treatment? If so, what should be used in the waters?

A-1. This should be taken to cause better eliminations. Have water body temperature, not hotter, not colder; and, as has been indicated, for each half gallon of water used—at first— put a level teaspoonful of table salt and half a teaspoonful of baking soda. In the last water put, to each gallon, a tablespoonful of Glyco-Thymoline—this the rinsing water. This will prevent the collapse to the body.   303-35

Q-8. Do I have any abnormal condition in my colon, and if so, what treatment should be given for same?

A-8. Well that every colon be cleansed occasionally with colonic irrigations. Here, naturally, when the blood supply has been contaminated and there is the tendency for the accumulations through the colon, this makes for some of the cells or pockets in same to at times carry, for too great a period, those fecal forces that become irritating and heavy. Hence once a month, or once in two months, or more often if necessary, use an irrigation; but be sure, particularly for this body, that there is carried in the water an antiseptic so that no irritation is produced. Or in the first portion of the water used, to each half gallon of water used add a level teaspoonful of salt—preferably iodized salt—and a heaping teaspoonful of baking soda, in the tepid water. In the last water as used, put a tablespoonful of Glyco-Thymoline to a quart of water, tepid.

This tends to leave an alkaline condition and yet is an antiseptic for the whole system.   843-2

For more information, consult the CF on Intestines: Constipation.

HONEYIDA WATER AND PLUTO WATER

Hunayadi (spelled Honeyida in the Cayce transcriptions) and Pluto water were two mineral salts, used as laxatives, which apparently are no longer available. Hunayadi water was a purgative mineral water of Hungarian (Cayce said Austrian) origin, named for the locality where it was obtained. Pluto water consisted of water to which magnesium sulphate (Epsom salts) and other minerals were added. The source of Pluto water was the French Lick Springs Hotel of French Lick, Indiana, and the water was occasionally referred to as French Lick water.

Hunayadi water was mentioned in readings for 14 individuals and Pluto water in readings for 12. Many readings mentioned them both, either finding them equally good options where a saline cathartic was needed or expressing a preference for one or the other. Alternatives mentioned in the readings include Epsom salts, Rochelle salts, Sal Hepatica and Eno salts.

ICHTHYOL

Ichthyol is a particular variety of the substance called Ichthammol, an ointment made by chemical breakdown and treatment of certain types of asphaltic rocks. This ointment is an antiseptic indicated for certain skin diseases. The readings recommended it about 25 times, particularly for bedsores and also in cases of eczema, dermatitis, pruritus (itching), and infections.

To a 23-year-old woman with scleroderma it was suggested she "Keep the Icthyol Ointment over those areas where there is the broken tissue, or where there are irritations." (2514-7)

INHALANT [2186-1]

In about 225 readings directions were given for formulating inhalants for all types of respiratory problems, including asthma, bronchitis, coughs, colds, emphysema, hay fever, pleurisy, pneumonia, post-nasal drip, sinusitis and tuberculosis. Depending on the condition involved, the formulas varied from case to case. Often this variation is so slight that many individuals find they can use different formulas interchangeably, with equally good results. The inhalant formula most widely used has been found, through research, to be one that can be generally recommended for almost any respiratory condition. This identical formula can be found in readings for asthma, hay fever and sinusitis, and similar versions were recommended for coughs and bronchitis.

Basically the inhalants recommended consist of pure grain alcohol to which small amounts of oils, such as oil of eucalyptus, rectified oil of turpentine, tincture of benzoin, tolu balsam, rectified creosote, and oil of pine needles have been added. Fumes arising from this solution are to be inhaled, as often as necessary for relief. Unlike most commercial decongestants on the market, the inhalants have no harmful side effects and there is no limit to how often they may be used. The fumes are most effective when used regularly several times a day.

The inhalant fumes function as an expectorant, meaning that they help the lungs and respiratory passages to expectorate or "slough off" excess mucus. The inhalant is also an antiseptic:

First we would prepare the inhalant, that there may be the antiseptic reaction from the gases for the throat, bronchials, lungs, that not only heal but that prevent accumulations from poor circulation through the muco-membranes of throat, nasal, bronchi, and the forces in the soft tissue of face, from becoming infected from these drosses. But it will aid also in keeping down the tendencies for the circulation to be so active through these portions.   421-8

. . .they [inhalant ingredients] will act not only as an antiseptic for the blood supply through the blood in and out through the body as it is inhaled, but will also be taken sufficient to act as an antiseptic through the intestinal system.
318-5

The following conditions are those in which inhalants were most often recommended.

Asthma:

. . .we would take in the system those properties [the

inhalant] that will help eliminate in the bloodstream and that will, through [the] respiratory system, give the better effect to the lungs and bronchials proper.   304-7

[Use the inhalant] to prevent the tickling sensation or the spasmodic condition occurring at times in the bronchials.
                                                                   304-3

Bronchitis:

. . .we would use a solution for cleansing or purifying the tissue that becomes involved. . .   837-1

As an inhalant to cleanse throat and bronchi of those disturbances that contribute to the upsetting of the liver and the digestive forces. . .   2975-1

Catarrh:
This term was formerly used for inflammation of mucous membranes, particularly those of the air passages of the nose and throat.

. . .we would use the inhalant that has been prescribed through these sources for the clarifying of the muco-membranes of head and throat. This would be inhaled, then, both through the nostril and into the throat, so that the glands of the throat and the muco-membranes in the tonsils, adenoid region, bronchi and lungs may all have that stimuli as to create constructive activity for these disturbed areas (or areas that become easily inflamed at times), reducing the tendency for the glands to overstimulate the muco-membranes and thus relieving the irritations. Not by the addition of stimulation in the circulation (that would disturb it) but by acting in the manner as an antiseptic that is penetrating in such a nature as to produce the proper balance in such tissue's activity in the system.   335-1

The purifying of the activities throughout the whole of the sympathetic forces, as from the clarifications of the breathing into the body those fumes (only, of course, the inhalations) will *strengthen* same. . .   826-1

Nasal Catarrh:

Also this will aid the activity of the kidneys and the circulation through the liver, that is naturally disturbed by the reflex condition of those poisons or congestions in the stomach itself.

See, the properties in the inhalant are also purifying to the body, to cleanse or to correct causes.   3094-1

This will tend to keep down those tendencies for acidity.
Q-1. What causes sore throat often and continuing for long periods?
A-1. As indicated, an irritation in the blood supply and the lymph as it flows through. The inhalant will aid in correcting this.   3107-1

Cold and Congestion:

Take as an inhalant—which will act as a blood stimulant, a blood clarifier, and in the form of a cleanser for the condition...   3987-1

[The inhalant] will overcome the tendencies for the body to be subject to cold and congestion.   687-1

Coughs:

The one [inhalant] for the cough and the bronchials [should be used], and that acts as an antiseptic for the prevention of tissue becoming involved by those of the bacilli as thrown off by the system attempting to *eliminate* through either respiratory or through the regular channel of the excretory functioning of the body.   4874-1

Hay Fever:

It will act upon the mucous membranes in such a way as to not only *prevent* the irritation but make bettered conditions in these directions.   808-8

As an antiseptic, and as a reducing agent to the plethoric condition caused in the passages of nose and throat themselves—for cold as well as for the acute conditions. . .
                   3180-1

Sinusitis:

[The inhalant should be used] when such radical changes are made, as in the atmospheric pressures, in the travel on train, or in closed or close offices, or the changes that make for these pressures on these portions of the system, especially when coming under the stress of a high mental activity of the body.
                   903-16

This will be found to be palliative and will prevent the *fullness* in the face and the throat. 600-1

Use this both as an inhalant and as a spray...for this, as will be found, is penetrating and will relieve those pressures in the soft tissue of the face and head circulation. 1131-2

...and we will find we can control the acidity or those tendencies for cold to affect the body. 2998-3

To use the inhalant as a spray, dilute a portion of the inhalant solution with two parts of distilled water. This is used in an atomizer, which may be purchased from a local drugstore.

For more information, consult the six CFs on lung problems, or the CFs on Catarrh: Nasal, Colds, Allergies, Hay Fever, Sinusitis, and Tuberculosis; also see in Dr. Reilly's book "The Common Cold."

Inhalant Ingredients:
Some of the inhalant ingredients mentioned in the readings are: tincture of benzoin, compound tincture of benzoin, Canadian balsam, oil of eucalyptus, oil of pine needles and tincture of tolu balsam. They are all natural and derived from plants. These substances, selected for use in the grain alcohol-based inhalants, have other uses as well.

A young woman of 24 years, suffering from hay fever, was told:

These properties [of the inhalant] are only antiseptics, but they tend to create through the sympathetic system an *effectual* preventative for this irritation. 934-2

Inhalant [261-8] was given for a man as a specific for his hay fever. It contained oil of eucalyptus, Canadian balsam, Benzosol, rectified creosote, tincture of benzoin, oil of turpentine, tolu in solution. Also see the CF on Hay Fever.

Oil of eucalyptus and oil of pine needles were recommended for use in fume baths, and can also be used in steam cabinets. Apparently there is benefit gained from the absorption by the skin of fumes arising from these oils. Fumes that are inhaled stimulate the lungs, acting as an expectorant and antiseptic. An effective vaporizer may be created by adding a few drops of these ingredients to a pan of steaming water. A little individual experimentation will determine which ingredients are most agreeable for this purpose.

An additional note from Gladys Davis: I use my favorite steam inhalant in the ordinary commercial vaporizer. It works fine! See reading 1208-9 in CF on Pneumonia. It is best to search the CFs and prepare your own inhalant as indicated in the case you select, or else have it prepared by a druggist as you need it.

INNERCLEAN

Innerclean is an herbal laxative compound containing agar, frangula, senna and psyllium seed. Its use was suggested in about 25 readings where improvement of the eliminations was indicated:

As to eliminants taken, we find that the vegetable compound would be much preferable for this body, especially to mineral salts or of that nature. Such then as Innerclean or the like would be the more preferable.   **464-23**

We would continue to keep an excess in eliminations. The Innerclean will be very satisfactory, if the [colonic] irrigations are used occasionally to prevent the Innerclean forming clogging conditions in the colon.   **849-63**

At times the readings cautioned against using such laxatives too frequently:

Q-5. Has Innerclean been harmful to this body?
A-5. At times it has. It tends to take too much of the lymph and emunctory circulation from the intestinal tract, or *dries* secretions without producing cleansing, taking away from the system the peristaltic movement or muscular contraction...
                                                                462-4

Q-6. Is it harmful to take Innerclean as a laxative every night?
A-6. This, under many or most conditions, is not harmful. In the present condition the body finds it rather irritating...
                                                                69-3

IODEX

Plain Iodex contains iodine in an ointment base. When in contact with skin abrasions the iodine is liberated by oxidation to prevent growth and action of bacteria and promote healing.

When applied on unbroken skin surfaces it is absorbed into the skin. This product was recommended about 13 times in the Cayce readings, in cases of boils, carbuncles, lymph tumors or cysts, dermatitis, bruises, eczema, and bedsores. Reading 522-4 stated that this was also an "applicant that takes soreness from bruised conditions."

For more information, consult the CF on Cancer: Skin.

IPANA TOOTHPASTE

Although the Ipana brand of toothpaste may actually still be on the market, the version recommended in 17 readings is no longer being made. This version of Ipana contained prickly ash bark, a substance which is particularly beneficial to the gums. A substitute toothpaste, however, now exists. Named Vicco, it contains 18 herbs intended to strengthen and invigorate the teeth and gums, including prickly ash bark. Vicco is blended according to the Ayurvedic science of India to prevent dental problems. This toothpaste and more information about it are available at some health food stores.

IPSAB [1800-34]

In about 70 Cayce readings a solution called Ipsab was recommended as a treatment for the gums and teeth. Many readings prescribing it also gave directions for making it, and these formulas varied somewhat in description from reading to reading. A few readings state that the finished product should be a paste, but the majority of readings refer to a liquid. If desired, a paste may be easily made by adding salt in sufficient amounts to the liquid.

The complete Ipsab formula contains prickly ash bark, salt, calcium chloride, peppermint and iodine. Salt acts as an astringent, shrinking the gum membranes between the teeth so that the other ingredients can reach these areas. The primary active ingredient is prickly ash bark. This was known to the American Indians as toothache bark, and the readings sometimes referred to it by the same term.

In many cases Ipsab was suggested simply for general upkeep of the teeth and gums:

Using, then for the teeth and gums, to strengthen same,

those properties as found in that combination as has been given for such conditions through these forces [Ipsab].

257-11

Some local attention [to the teeth] is needed. The natural tendency of a disturbance in the circulatory forces to the sensory organs, as indicated, is to make for a lack of the proper circulation through the gums and to the portions of the teeth themselves.

If the solution known as Ipsab is used to massage the gums occasionally, it will make for a *strengthening* of the areas and a preserving of their usefulness. Once or twice a week this would be thoroughly massaged into the gums, and will make a great deal of change in the gums and the teeth. Do that.

987-1

Do use Ipsab as a massage for the gums and it will make a great deal of difference with the teeth, the breath and the general activity.

3598-1

We would use same [Ipsab] not upon cotton, for this body, but upon the finger use it and massage; not only the gums where the teeth are but where they are not! And we will find that the stimulation to the activities of the throat itself, to the salivary glands, to even the tonsil area, will be materially aided by the activity of the combination of the calcium with the iodine in same, as well as the antiseptics that arise from the vegetable forces in same as combined with sodium chloride. 569-23

Ipsab was recommended for the developing teeth of babies, applied in diluted form. The following readings were given for a one-year-old and a nine-month-old child, respectively:

Also during this period of the formation of the teeth, keep sufficient quantities of iodine in the food values for the body, as well as calcium and so forth. It will be found that a massage of the gums occasionally with those properties known as Ipsab will be helpful in making for a healthy condition as these processes are carried on through the activity of the thyroid operations in the body.

314-2

Q-2. Are teeth forming normally?
A-2. These are very good. We would find that a weakened solution of Ipsab for the gums would tend to relieve the pressure and make for normalcy in the salivary glands, as well as strengthening the tissue [in the] mouth. This should be reduced at least half, and the gums massaged with a tuft of cotton with same. This also adds to the amount of saline,

calcium and iodine, for the activity of the glands in mouth and throat.   299-2

Ipsab seems to be especially effective in treatment of bleeding or receding gums and for treatment and prevention of pyorrhea. One reading stated that some element in the prickly ash bark destroyed the "germs" that cause pyorrhea. Ipsab was also advised in one case of trenchmouth and in other types of gum problems:

Q-1. What can I do about pyorrhea condition in my teeth?
A-1. Use Ipsab regularly each day and rinse mouth out when it is finished with Glyco-Thymoline.   5121-1

The receding gums and those tendencies towards pyorrhea would be allayed by the consistent use of Ipsab as a massage for the teeth and gums. Also these should be treated, some locally, with the dentist's paraphernalia—[as well as] the small wads of cotton saturated with the Ipsab and applied in the areas where the conditions are indicated at the base or edge of the gums.   3696-1

This will *purify* and make for such a condition as to assist in correcting the trouble where there has been the softening of the teeth themselves—or the enamel on same.   1026-1

It will not only relieve these conditions [infection at root of teeth] but be helpful for the whole general system.   325-55

We would have some local attention to the teeth and gums. We would use the preparation of Ipsab for the hardening and toughening of the gums, cleansing also the teeth with same will make for better conditions; but this would be preferably done after there has been the local attention to some of these that need it, because—of course—the application of the properties in Ipsab does not heal broken [dentine] or the enamel or where exposed nerves are shown; though with its application it'll *prevent* tooth decay, for it will cleanse the disorders that make for the reaction and keep the condition more alkaline in this area.   514-4

As in the above reading, Ipsab was often suggested in combination with regular professional care of the teeth. Sometimes the readings stated that drastic measures such as removal of teeth could be avoided if Ipsab was used prior to visiting the dentist:

This [root canal work] will be locally very good. But as we find, if there will be the suggested treatments followed for the *general* condition of the body, and a local application of those properties combined in the compound known as Ipsab—used as a massage, *much* of this condition with the teeth would be relieved without so *much* local attention. And we would find the mouth in much better condition for such work to be carried out, than in the immediate future.   1101-4

Q-4. Should the body have the teeth taken out?
A-4. Rather would we use, with the corrections of the system [osteopathic], those properties of the Ipsab as a massage for these. Then, as the centralization comes, and defective conditions are to be met, these would be *locally* treated—not take them out as yet.   307-2

In addition to its use for massage, Ipsab can also be used as a mouthwash:

Use Ipsab as a good mouth massage and rinse. Massage the gums with this first and then rinse the mouth with it. Do this once or twice a week.   3902-1

Dietary advice sometimes accompanied Ipsab recommendations. One reading stated that anyone using Ipsab should eat a salad of raw vegetables every day.

On Oct. 17, 1972, Gladys Davis made this notation under the 1800-1 report: An article on Ipsab appearing in the November, 1972, issue of *The A.R.E. Journal* by Tom Johnson and Carol A. Baraff states, "It is not known where the name originated." This reminds me to make this notation. The name was suggested by Gertrude Cayce, combining the first letters of the main ingredients: Iodine, Peppermint, Salt and Prickly Ash Bark.

For more information, consult the CFs on Teeth: Pyorrhea and Baby Care.

JERUSALEM ARTICHOKES

One individual was told in a reading that eating one hen's-egg-sized (two to three ounces) Jerusalem artichoke a week would be good for everyone if eaten in season (fall through spring). They were often recommended for improving the activity of the assimilations and eliminations, and were suggested in most cases of diabetes as an effective and beneficial alternative to insulin injections. Children were to be given artichokes that were smaller than the hen's egg size recommended for adults to avoid overstimulation of the pancreas. Various readings also advised against eating pickled artichokes or artichokes prepared with vinegar, and products made with artichoke flour.

Jerusalem artichokes can be served raw in salad or cooked. Some readings advised alternating their manner of preparation in this way. If cooked, the artichokes should preferably be prepared in Patapar Paper (vegetable parchment), as many readings advised. This method preserves valuable juices which should be eaten along with each cooked artichoke. A little butter and salt can be used as seasoning. If water is used in cooking, it is advisable to drink this liquid afterward.

If it is impractical to store the artichokes in the ground as recommended, they will keep best stored in the refrigerator, in potting soil or peat moss. In spring they have a tendency to sprout, but may of course be eaten while in the sprouting stage.

For more information consult the CF on Diabetes.

KALDAK

Kaldak was a nutritional supplement recommended in about 80 readings, primarily in cases of general debilitation and also for anemia, arthritis and poor assimilations. The readings suggested its use as a tonic to increase the number of red blood cells by supplying iron, phosphates, silicon, and B-complex vitamins to the system. Apparently, Kaldak was made available in at least two forms, both sources of the above nutrients. One consisted of a debittered "chip type" brewers yeast fortified with vitamin D and phosphorus. Another was a liquid said to contain liver, vitamin B-1, niacin and iron. This product was made by the KalDak Company in Lansing, Michigan. The manufacturers recommended its use as an all-purpose supplement, for general body building as well as conditions such as arthritis, neuritis, nervousness, colitis, constipation, chronic fatigue, run down condition, digestive distress, gastro-intestinal disorders, etc. A possible substitute is a Vitamin B Complex Syrup with Iron.

LAXATIVE CAPSULES [294-12]

This combination of four laxative herbs resembles—

sometimes closely—at least 110 other similar preparations found in the readings. The number of ingredients in these preparations ranges from two to six in various combinations and proportions. The formula given in reading 294-12 contains the four most frequently mentioned herbs: podophyllin (mandrake), licorice, cascara sagrada and black root (leptandrin). Other herbs included less frequently in such formulas were sanguinaria and senna.

This particular formula was given for Cayce himself, who at the time was suffering from hypertension (high blood pressure), impaired liver functioning and poor metabolism. The reading commented that the preparation would equalize the excretory and secretive functioning of the liver, resulting in an equalization of the circulation, hence lowering the blood pressure. Similar formulas were given in a wide range of conditions, typically involving poor assimilations and eliminations, including at least one other case of hypertension.

The instructions in this reading were simply to take three capsules. Other readings gave varying dosages, such as daily for five days, every other day until three, five or ten are taken, or once every third day or every week. Sometimes evening dosage was specified.

See CFs on pertinent conditions such as Liver: Torpid and Sinusitis. There are many CFs on different ailments advising various combinations of these ingredients, depending on the individual need (as in case 341-43 on sinusitis, etc.). Before having the druggist prepare the combinations for you, be sure your physician advises it for you in the right proportions and dosage suitable in your case.

LIQUID LANOLIN

Lanolin is a substance secreted by the hair follicles of sheep, and is derived from the wool. Lanolin in liquid form was recommended in about 165 readings as an ingredient in a variety of massage and lotion formulas—though never by itself. It is included in the formulas for Massage Formula [1968-7] (formerly Aura Glow/Rose Petals), and Scar Formula [2015-10] (formerly Scarmassage Scar Formula), and Arthritis Massage Formula [3363-1] (formerly Egyptian Balm Arthritis Liniment).

According to reading 2768-1, lanolin acts soothingly in combination with other oils, thus preventing them from irritating the skin.

If it burns too much, or produces irritation, then add ½ teaspoonful of lanolin to the solution, see?   2768-1

Often the readings called for dissolved lanolin. Either melted, emulsified lanolin or lanolin oil (lanolin with wax removed) may be used.

For more information consult the appropriate CFs on Arthritis, Complexion and Scars.

LIMEWATER

Limewater is a saturated solution of slaked lime (calcium hydroxide) in water, used as an antacid. Limewater contains calcium, and was often mentioned in readings for babies and children as an aid in developing strong teeth and bones. It may be added to water following nursing or other feeding, or added to milk or juice.

Q-3. Any special care to keep teeth strong and healthy?
A-3. Give her a little Calcios or limewater.   2752-3

Q-2. How much limewater should be used at a time?
A-2. Half a teaspoonful to a pint of milk or to a cup of the juice.   305-1

It will be necessary for the modifying of the food, or milk, that is given the body [baby, three weeks old, suffering from colic].

But, as we find, it would be more helpful to add a teaspoonful of limewater to each quantity of milk as nursed, see? Necessarily this would be diluted; not put in the milk but diluted and given afterwards. . .

Q-5. For the hiccoughing [what is cause and cure]?
A-5. This is natural, and—with the limewater—will be eliminated.   928-1

Limewater added with the milk will "carry more vitamin D in the system. We do not want to *over*balance, or to cause an extraordinary growth to any glands that would tend to make for extremes in the developing body. These [limewater] added in overabundance aid, add to, those glands which produce unusual activities in these directions." (299-2)

For more information, consult the CF on Baby Care.

MASSAGE FORMULA [1968-7]

In reading 1968-7 a formula was given for a general skin lotion that had some interesting claims made for it:

This will not only keep a stimulating [effect]. . .taken occasionally, and give the body a good base for the stimulating of the superficial circulation; but [the solution] will aid in keeping the *body beautiful;* that is, as to [being free from] any blemish of any nature. 1968-7

The original formula given in this reading contained peanut oil, olive oil, lanolin, and rosewater. Unfortunately, natural rosewater spoils easily, and when in combination with oils it appears to cause the oils to grow rancid more quickly. If following the reading precisely, therefore, it is preferable to mix the ingredients for a short time usage.

The peanut oil/olive oil/lanolin combination is the most typical massage formulation in the readings. Of all oils mentioned in the readings they are the most frequently recommended. Peanut oil massages were often suggested for the prevention of arthritis and for the supplying of energies to the body, as in 1158-31. Another reading stated that:

. . .if these [massages] are kept consistently, we will not only build strength but supply the better circulation throughout the whole body. 1688-7

See the CF on Complexion; also in Dr. Reilly's book, "Cayce Massage Mixtures" and "Beauty Problems."

MAYPOP BITTERS [543-5]

An infusion (water extract) of the passion flower herb *(Passiflora incarnata),* also variously known as Maypop, Mayflower, or Mayblossom Bitters, was often recommended for epilepsy in the Cayce readings. A fusion is made basically by simmering the dried herb (or fresh when possible) in water and then adding sufficient alcohol to preserve it. Apparently at one time a version of this formula was commercially available, and some readings recommended it. Many others offered directions for making it.

Passion flower has a sedative effect on the system with the great advantage that it is non-habit-forming. Reading 4844-3 states that there will be no drug-forming habit resulting from the use of this kind of sedative. Often the passion flower fusion is given as a substitute for other sedatives, such as Phenobarbitol and Dilantin, which may have undesirable side effects.

In the general stress some conditions show some aggravation as respecting *impulses*. This from lack of amount of sedative active forces in [the] system, with [the] changes as taking place. Be well were those properties of the Maypop or passion flower, made in *this* proportion and manner, given to the body, see? Then we will find we will be able to diminish the amount of those sedative forces that so choke portions of the blood supply in its capillary circulation, especially—and be more helpful in the general conditions of the body.   543-5

In the following reading precautions regarding diet, while this is being taken, are also advised:

In the general considering of the conditions of the body in the present, for the better conditions, we will find that the use of the Mayblossom Bitters—taken properly—will be much more beneficial than those of the more active sedative natures; for the herbs in Mayblossom Bitters act with the system—especially the nitre or saltpeter that is given in small quantities to retard those reactions for the contraction of muscular forces in [the] system—better than the Luminol or any of the Bromides. These [Mayblossom Bitters], then, may be reduced somewhat in the quantity, but taken oftener—so that three to four, even five teaspoonsful, may be taken during 24 hours—see? but if these are taken, and there is congestion through [the] digestive system—through improper diet—they will only irritate, rather than aid.   543-7

The best general guideline to follow, if additional sedatives must be used, is to avoid taking them on the same days that the passion flower is taken, unless directed otherwise by a doctor. One individual who began taking passion flower fusion also began to experience more frequent attacks. The readings attributed this to the taking of other sedatives at the same time and commented:

These [properties in passion flower compound] have apparently produced greater spasmodic frequency. This was to be expected, when there have been those activities under the sedatives to allay same. For, these are as two natures within the system warring one against another; both active upon the same atomic influences within the activity of this portion of the body itself.   2153-6

Other readings offer more information on the effect of passion flower on the system—particularly the nerves:

. . .the Maypop is for the nerve system and for the blood supply, as is hindered by the improper incentives through the connection between the glands at the base of the brain and the hypogastric nerve center, which governs the digestion and the assimilation in portions of the system. . .   4678-1

The passion flower effect is upon the sympathetic nervous system. It is to relinquish the congestions that are produced in the attacks of incoordination at the base of the brain, through the flexure as indicated which is produced through the areas along the spine, and in the adhesions in the area indicated.
                                                            2153-5

The reaction of these is to the pyloric and the activities of the glandular systems within the functioning of the lacteals, about the gall duct area itself.   2153-6

Dosage advised varied from three to five teaspoonsful daily, with dosage reduced proportionately for children. Whatever amount is decided upon should be taken consistently in regular cycles. It may be advisable to reduce dosage during the female menstrual cycle:

Those administrations for the changes in the glands in the system will be more effective [if these will] be given so that they coincide with the active forces in [the] system as respecting the menstrual periods. These, as we find, would be best given, then, more of an *orderly* nature; that is, more in quantity and more in active forces just after and just preceding the periods, and not so *much* during that ten-day interim, as is seen. This will prevent too much of same being active with the lymphatic circulation.   543-3

When taken consistently passion flower fusion can apparently be instrumental in helping to reduce symptoms of epilepsy, and sometimes eliminate them entirely. At this point a reduced dosage may be continued, or dosage may be discontinued to be resumed only if the need is felt. One individual was told that he would have to take five gallons before he was finished with the treatment, and the attacks had completely ceased:

Now, in a preparation as will eliminate the attacks entirely, prepare as this: Because the attacks are farther apart, or because they are eliminated to where they become minor in nature do not stop.   1001-10

Most formulations of passion flower fusion include wild ginseng, "that is—according to the ancients—the basis of the stimulation of life in its very essence in the body of man." (636-1)

For more information consult the CF on Epilepsy.

It is recommended that you consult a physician before using this product.

MULLEIN

Mullein is an herb recommended about fifteen times in the readings. According to the Cayce source it can be particularly valuable taken as a tea for cases of varicose veins. Either the fresh or the dry herb may be used, although whichever is chosen, it should be taken consistently. If the fresh is in season, this is perhaps preferable, although the following reading advises the dry for the sake of uniformity:

Take internally mullein tea not more than three times a week, but make it fresh each time it is taken. Prepare a tea made from mullein. For uniformity, preferably use the dry mullein, a pinch between thumb and forefinger. Put into a teacup and pour boiling water on same. Let this stand for 30 minutes, strain, cool and drink. This is a reaction to the liver, the lungs, the heart and the kidneys, as to produce coordinating activity in circulation. It works with each of these and also makes a better condition through the alimentary canal.   5148-1

We would also take mullein tea. This should be made of the fresh, green, tender leaves. Pour a pint of boiling water over an ounce of the mullein leaves and let steep for about 20 to 30 minutes. Then strain and keep in the ice box, so that it may be kept fresh. Take about an ounce to an ounce and a half of this each day. Make this fresh at least every two or three days. Keep this up, and it will aid in the circulation, in the elimination of the character of acid in the system, and aid in the circulation through the veins—that are disturbing.
                                    243-38

If there will be the walking, and not merely standing or resting, and the taking of a small quantity of mullein tea every other day, these [swellings in the limbs caused by pregnancy] will disappear—and this disturbance will disappear. The therapeutic reaction is to better circulation—through the kidneys, especially as related to the lower limbs.   457-13

This taken occasionally is not bad for anybody and it will be very good for you.   457-14

In one reading, for an individual with a skin rash caused by poor eliminations, directions were given for making a mullein tonic. For those who find it is too much trouble to make the tea fresh every few days, the tonic is probably a good alternative, since with addition of the grain alcohol it will keep indefinitely.

Mullein leaves can also be used in the form of stupes or poultices. In some cases of varicose veins this application was recommended in addition to taking the tea internally. Stupes are prepared and utilized as follows, using green leaves if available:

Gather the mullein leaves, bruise these and pour boiling water over them (in an enamel pan or glass container, not aluminum or tin). Then place over the affected areas. 5037-1

We would apply the mullein stupes now more to those areas that are the *sources* from which the limbs receive their circulatory activity, and those portions about the limb to reduce the swelling. Apply these about once a day, and for about an hour.   1541-6

Mullein stupes are useful in cases of kidney stones as well. The readings claim that this can help to dissolve the stones themselves:

Or, there may be alternated with same [turpentine packs], to relax the body more, the mullein stupes. Crush the leaves and apply between gauze, you see, over the area. We will find healing from these, as well as the inclination for the dissolving or breaking up of the stone by the absorption.   843-6

Frequency of application depends upon the severity of the condition.

For more information, consult the CFs on Blood Vessels: Varicose Veins and Kidneys: Stones.

MUSCLE AND BRUISE LINIMENT

A massage formula given in reading 326-5 has come into wide usage in treatment of backaches, sprains, strained muscles and ligaments, bruises and related problems. The formula contains olive oil, Nujol, witch hazel, tincture of benzoin, oil of sassafras and coal oil (kerosene).

It'll be necessary to shake this together for it will tend to separate; but a small quantity massaged in the cerebrospinal system or over sprains, joints, swellings, bruises will *take out* the inflammation or pain! 326-5

This same massage formula was also recommended for varicose veins:

And we will find that the massage of the compound that has been given for bruises, strains, and such conditions for the body, would be most helpful for this particular body also. Use same from the lower dorsal all the way to the lower portion of the feet, down the limbs, across the abdomen and especially down the side of the thigh where the veins are, and over the calf or lower portion of the limbs, showing dilation and swelling so much. 243-18

Rapid healing of affected areas can be promoted with greater effectiveness if heat is applied following application of the oils.

In many cases involving massage, the readings suggested shaking the oils together thoroughly, then pouring no more than the amount to be used into a saucer and dipping the fingers into this solution. The purpose of this practice is to avoid possible contamination of the original solution from bacteria on the skin surface.

For more information consult the CF on Fractures and Sprains; also see in Dr. Reilly's book "Cayce Massage Mixtures."

MYRRH TINCTURE AND OLIVE OIL

Myrrh tincture is an alcoholic solution containing myrrh, which is an extract of gum resin from trees in the Red Sea coastal forests. A few readings suggested it for internal use, but it was most often recommended in combination with olive oil, for massage.

...tincture of myrrh acts with the pores of the skin in such a manner as to strike in, causing the circulation to be carried to affected parts [scars, in this case]...   440-3

Reading 618-4 stated that myrrh was good for the muscles and would stimulate the superficial circulation.

A trade name, *Myr-Plus,* formulated some years ago by an A.R.E. member and Cooperating Physician, contains myrrh and peanut oil. He found that this combination could be kept indefinitely, while the myrrh and olive oil combination would separate and had to be made fresh every two to three days.

The trade name *Myrola* is a new combination of myrrh and olive oil which, it is claimed, will keep as long as other massage preparations.

If following the readings precisely, it is preferable to mix the ingredients for home use exactly as described:

Heat the olive oil to add the myrrh, not to boiling but nearly so, and add the myrrh. About a tablespoonful of each should be used. This [would be] the quantity to be used at each application...   5467-1

See in Dr. Reilly's book "Cayce Massage Mixtures"; also see the CFs in which they were recommended.

OLIVE OIL SHAMPOO

Olive Oil Shampoo was recommended about ten times in the Cayce readings, making it the most frequently recommended type of shampoo. Olive Oil Shampoo and Castile Shampoo are often similar, and sometimes in the readings these terms are used interchangeably. No particular brand was ever recommended, although in one reading it was stressed that any brand of shampoo chosen should be "pure."

In some readings Olive Oil Shampoo was simply suggested without explanation:

Use a good cleansing agent for the scalp, with a good tonic afterward—Olive Oil Shampoo would be well for this body.
3517-1

Other readings suggest that the olive oil is beneficial to the scalp:

For this particular body, use Olive Oil Shampoo, for there is needed the oil for the scalp and the opening of [the pores of]

same. Cleanse the scalp with some good cleanser, preferably [Packer's?] Tar Soap, and then apply the Olive Oil Shampoo.
3379-1

As for wash, preferably this would be done with those *oils*— rather than acids or alkalines. Such as an Olive Oil Shampoo, using as the cleanser for same that of the pure Castile soap, or Castile with a little tar soap in same. Be sure that this is *rinsed* well from hair and scalp.
255-10

Plain Castile is the *best* to be used. Castile Shampoo, see, will add a lustre—of course, would be well if a few drops of olive *oil* is added in the water, not in the hair.
658-2

Olive Oil Shampoo was also advised several times in conjunction with crude oil, white Vaseline and 20% grain alcohol for treatment and prevention of baldness:

Take at least five to ten minutes to massage the scalp with the white petroleum jelly. Afterwards take an Olive Oil Shampoo.
970-1

As for this particular condition, it arises from a poor circulation. Once a week we would wash the hair with a very *pure* soap (preferably the purest, which is Castile). Then massage into the scalp very small quantities of the white Vaseline, each time after the shampoo. The next day clarify same with a twenty percent (20%) solution of alcohol; *grain* alcohol, not wood or denatured. These used, as we find, will make for the better conditions; and will tend to make for the natural curl, the natural texture and strength of the hair itself.
852-13

And, for cosmetic purposes, this advice was given:

Q-12. How can I best care for my hair and keep it light, and from turning dark at the roots?
A-12. Use an Olive Oil Shampoo. This as we find would be the better way. Shampoo it at least once each week.
1431-2

For more information, consult the CFs on Complexion and Hair.

PATAPAR PAPER
(Now called Vegetable Parchment)

Patapar Paper is a non-toxic, tasteless and odorless sheet of specially processed paper, which is grease-resistant and keeps its strength when wet. In readings advising the inclusion of cooked vegetables in the diet, Patapar Paper was often recommended for use in cooking. By this method vegetables are tied in a dampened sheet of this paper and placed in simmering water until done. Apparently this method aids in the retention of valuable vitamins and minerals:

...cook most of the vegetables in Patapar Paper, preserving their own juices and serving them in their own juices...
3033-1

The vegetables that are taken should be preferably cooked in their *own* juices, as in Patapar Paper. This will make a vast difference in the building of resistance.   861-1

There are certain vegetables that, with the processes in Patapar Paper, the mineral salts which are most active with the human body are preserved.   1158-38

Q-4. What foods or treatments are especially good for bringing more of the luster—reds, coppers, and golds—back into the hair?
A-4. Nothing better than the peelings of Irish potatoes or the juices from same. Don't just put the peelings in water and cook them, because most of the necessary properties will go out, but put them in Patapar Paper to cook them.   2072-14

Each day with the evening meal take one ounce of beet juice, from cooked beets—but cooked in their *own* juice, as in Patapar Paper, and using only the juice that comes from same. They may be cut and placed in the Patapar Paper, for this will allow more of the juice to be released.   2207-1

PINE TAR SHAMPOO AND SOAP

Pine tar soap was mentioned in about seven readings. In every case it was the soap that was recommended—not the shampoo—although in all of these cases it was to be applied to the scalp as a shampoo. It is possible that only the soap was being made in Cayce's day, and that the shampoo did not appear on the market until later. A specific brand of tar soap was mentioned in one reading:

Q-8. What soap should be used for washing [the hair and scalp—following crude oil application]?
A-8. The better is Packer's Tar, for the *general* use.
275-30

Because of the antiseptic nature of the pine oil contained in the pine tar soap, its use was most often indicated for scalp treatments, in conjunction with such items as white Vaseline, Olive Oil Shampoo, crude oil and diluted grain alcohol.

Case 261-2, the reading most commonly followed for dandruff, involves application of diluted grain alcohol mixed with a small amount of pine oil, followed by white Vaseline and a thorough cleansing of the head with tar soap.

[To] keep it [the hair] nice and smooth. Take care of it more often with either Drene Hair Tonic or olive oil hair tonic, followed with the shampooing with crude oil and tar soap...These, while making irritation at first will maintain the better conditions for the body. **5261-1**

For the scalp [dryness] and for the hair, we find it would be well to have a thorough massage or shampoo with pure tar soap—at least once a week, and then to massage a little white Vaseline into the scalp after such a shampoo. This will materially aid the hair and produce a better condition there. **633-12**

RADIO-ACTIVE APPLIANCE or IMPEDANCE DEVICE

An appliance, referred to at various times by the terms Radio-Active Appliance and Impedance Device, was mentioned about 455 times in the readings. Actually there is nothing radio-active about this device, at least not in today's atomic age connotations for this term. It is possible that the vibrational current theoretically produced between the Appliance and the body of the user is in some way analogous to or comparable to a radio wave.

The Radio-Active Appliance is a battery for the construction of which the readings supplied details. By itself it does not generate any measurable electrical energy, although it seems to affect the electrical energies of the body. The readings recommend its use particularly to improve the circulation and normalize the functioning of the nervous system; thus it aids in relaxing the body. It was given as more of a preventative than a cure for serious physical disorders, although cases in which the Appliance was suggested include the following, in order of frequency: nervous tension and incoordination, circulation, coordination, insomnia, neurasthenia, debilitation, hypertension, abnormal children, deafness, obesity, and arthritis.

The readings often commented that the plain Radio-Active Appliance would be beneficial for almost anyone, so long as instructions for proper usage were observed. In special cases, for curative purposes, a solution jar containing various substances, such as gold chloride, silver nitrate, tincture of iron, spirits of camphor, tincture of iodine or Atomidine*, was to be attached to the Appliance for the purpose of transmitting certain needed elements from these solutions vibratorially into the system. Apparently the effect of the solution in the circuit is to stimulate the system to produce the needed elements; the solution does not actually enter the body. An example of this application would be the use of tincture of iron in cases of anemia or tincture of iodine for goitre. The effect of these solutions on the body is even more of a mystery than the theory behind the Appliance itself. A metallurgist has theorized that the solutions, when separated into positive and negative ions, might alter the current in the Appliance as an audio signal modulates a radio carrier wave.

A great deal of additional material on the construction and use of the Radio-Active Appliance is available. See the CF on Appliances: Radio-Active (Impedance Device) and the A.R.E. booklet on the electrical appliances described in the Edgar Cayce readings. Rather than repeating this information, we quote here some readings' extracts regarding the effect of the Appliance on the body:

[The Radio-Active Appliance is not electrical in the accepted sense; it] *uses the electricity of the body* to equalize the circulation. **2344-5**

. . .the lowest form of electrical vibration *is* the basis of life. The application of such vibrations to the body when it is fagged in mind, in physical endurance, will stimulate the necessary influences for the body to return to the abilities within self to carry on. . . **444-2**

[The] Radio-Active Appliance [is] good for *anyone,* especially for those that tire or need an equalizing of the circulation, which is necessary for anyone that uses the brain a great deal, or that is unactive on the feet as much as is sufficient to keep the proper circulation. **826-3**

. . .coordinating of the physical body with the mental body

---

*It is recommended that you consult a physician before using this product.

creates that which is commonly known as memory. An assistance to this will be found in the use of the Radio-Active Appliance, which is well for everyone and especially good with this body. . .if we will allow a perfect physical body to coordinate with the activities about it, it *creates* a memory.

416-9

The Appliance balances the vibratory rate in the extremities in the system (body complex).

Those vibrations from the Appliance given are not just as talismanic conditions, nor are they that which operates through the imaginations of a body, but when *properly compounded* or constructed these correspond with the laws of physics and of elemental forces. . .for building in a physical manner. While they are seemingly of little or no use from outward appearance. . .those laws [are implemented] that replenish through continuity of vibratory rates built or created in various portions of the system, and equalized through that vibration sent out. This enables the quieting, then, from within, and allows the forces to become predominant that are constructive to *vitality* in [the] system.

957-3

Equalizing of circulation to its normal condition, forcing coordination by the nerve reaction in [the] system and relieving congestion in any portion of [the] body. . .may occur at that time [the Appliance is used], bringing the better normal sleep to [the] body, giving the physical forces the opportunity for recuperation through the equalized circulation.   538-12

. . .*whenever* there are the periods of overtiredness, overanxiety, the desire on the part of the body to make for *real* rest, use same. . .   1022-1

Q-8. How often and how much longer should [the] Radio-Active Appliance be used?

A-8. If it is *not* to the advantage of the body in that it gives an opportunity for the use of its spiritual balance, leave it off! For it can be made very detrimental!

But if it is used at the period for the body to meditate and pray, thus making a better coordination between all of its *mental* and *spiritual* and *physical* forces, the longer it is used the better! Not at one period, of course, but continuously over a long period, for the whole of the mental and spiritual and physical reactions.

This is beneficial to *anyone, properly* used! It is harmful, improperly used.

You can't use the Radio-Active Appliance and be a good "cusser" or "swearer"—neither can you use it and be a good hater. For it will work as a boomerang to the whole of the nervous system if used in conjunction with such an attitude.

It is the coordinating effect of the balancing powers in the nervous system, as related to the mental and physical and spiritual bodies, that becomes active with the use of such an Appliance. 1844-2

We will find that impulse [from the Appliance, used with gold], whether as to that of senility when produced from old age alone or senility as produced by conditions produced in the brain itself; for *with* the proper manipulations to *produce* coordination *with* drainage in the system, as may be given through manipulation osteopathically, or neuropathically given to the system under various stages, may create for a body almost a new brain, will the patience, the suggestion, the activities in the system *be* carried out. . . 1800-16

. . .we find this, as has been given, would prove very beneficial in any condition relating to the vibratory forces in [the] physical body, especially that of first stages of rheumatism, catarrh, or any condition that affects the system regarding the elimination for the body.

This we find would be well that everyone use such an Appliance, for the system would be improved in every condition that relates to the body being kept in attunement. . . 1800-5

This will relieve that tendency of cold feet, that tendency of poor circulation in the extremities. . . 326-1

The use of the Radio-Active Appliance keeps nearer the normalcy as to weight, if any pressures are removed along the cerebrospinal system. This would be true for most anybody. . . 877-18

By adding vibrations from the Radio-Active Appliance (the plain), the assimilated forces would be better distributed in the system and. . .will act with the glands of the system that tend to make for too much of the avoirdupois [weight] of the body. 2096-2

There are about 200 readings recommending the use of the Radio-Active Appliance at a time when the patient can be quiet and in a meditative state. In addition to case 1844-2, which appeared earlier, here is another reference mentioning that particular use.

During such application [of the Radio-Active Appliance] the body should be in that position of [being] retrospective within itself, as to that as may be accomplished *within* self *through* the application of *concentration* in self...the manipulations at least twice each week for two to three weeks, then *rest* [from them] two to three weeks and take another course of treatments or adjustments—but keep *up* those [periods] of the concentration; that is, entering into the silence with self, and [in?] those vibrations from the Radio-Active Appliance. 10-1

It is recommended that you consult a physician before using this product.

RADIUM APPLIANCES

Readings for approximately 160 individuals recommended a type of therapy which made use of the healing properties of the radioactive element radium. The devices recommended for this purpose were known as the Radium Appliance, available in regular or double strength, and Degnen's Lens. The Appliance was a pad which was wrapped around the body, usually over the solar plexus area, and could be worn during the day, at night, or both, as needed. The Lens was a set of goggles which were worn over the eyes as a treatment for blindness and other eye disorders. Both were charged with radium, and the Appliance could be recharged for a period of time by placing it regularly in strong sunlight.

These and several other devices were manufactured by the Radium Appliance Company, located in Los Angeles, which termed itself the maker of "Degnen's Solar Seal Brand Radio-Active Therapeutical Appliances and Preparations." Riding the crest of radium's popularity as a cure-all in the early part of this century, the company apparently did a thriving business for a time, but is now no longer in existence.

Radium is still used medically today in the treatment of cancer and some skin disorders, but both Cayce and the manufacturers of the device had a much broader concept of its uses. The Cayce readings recommended the Appliance for a broad spectrum of disorders, most notably general debilitation, as well as eye problems, spinal subluxations, toxemia, some types of cancer, and ulcers. The readings recommended it to build the blood, rejuvenate the nerves, and raise the vibrations:

In this body, then, the higher vibrations as would be found in the Radium Appliance, that gives new life, new blood supply to

93

the physical forces of the body—creating a perfect coordination throughout the physical; thus allowing the mental and spiritual forces to manifest in the body.   4735-1

The manufacturers held a remarkably similar view of their Appliance's capacities, although they recommended it for everyone, where Cayce did not. A letter to Cayce from their sales manager went into some detail about its benefits to the nerves, bloodstream and circulation, concluding: "We find there are practically no conditions of ill health that are not favorably affected by this radio-active treatment when given a fair trial." (2646-6 Supplement)

It should be noted that the Radium Appliance is not the same as radium water, which was recommended to 14 individuals in treatment of cancer and various other disorders. This was obtained from the Radium Water Company in Pittsburgh and there is no known substitute for it today.

RAGWEED LAXATIVE [369-12]

Ragweed, also known as ambrosia weed, received mention by Cayce in more than 125 formulas. It was recommended in most instances as a tonic and as a laxative, and also as an aid in both the assimilating and eliminating processes, as in the following quotation:

Will there be taken in the system, at regular intervals, those properties that are not habit-forming, neither are they effective towards creating the condition where cathartics are necessary for the activities through the alimentary canal— whether related to the colon or the jejunum, or ileum—yet these will change the vibrations in such a manner as to keep clarified the assimilations, and aid the pancreas, the spleen, the liver and the hepatic circulation, in keeping a normal equilibrium. These properties would be found in those of the ambrosia weed. . .This will aid the digestive system, will aid the whole of the *eliminating* system.   454-1

The readings frequently mentioned that ragweed was beneficial as a laxative because it was non-habit-forming and did not cause the body to develop a dependence on laxatives. Various ragweed formulations were given as substitutes for a product called Simmons Liver Regulator, now off the market, also a laxative. Some versions of these compounds described in the readings contained only ragweed, simple syrup and grain alcohol, while others included additional ingredients, such as balsam of tolu, syrup of sarsaparilla and licorice. The Liver Regulator itself contained ragweed and licorice. Sometimes the readings offered reasons for this substitution:

Where this [Liver Regulator] is given for anyone, the better preparation would be to make it out of the ragweed, which is the basis of same—either the green (but dry same) or the dry, which may be preserved or bought in bulk, and made in the form of a tea...[The reading then described how the dried herb should be simmered in distilled water, with grain alcohol then added.]

And you have better than Simmons Liver Regulator for activity on the liver! This for anyone! This is the *best* of the vegetable compounds for activities of the liver. Of course, if made commercially we would add some few other things to it.
369-12

Perhaps by "other things" the reading was referring to the sarsaparilla, licorice and balsam of tolu recommended in combination with ragweed in reading 304-18, which also described a substitute for the Liver Regulator.

The Cayce source must have foreseen that the Simmons Liver Regulator would go off the market, which it did many years later but not during his lifetime.

Ragweed also has other uses. It was indicated as a preventative for appendicitis:

If the most hated of the weeds were used [green] as a portion of the diet it would never occur. . .   644-1

Reading 349-20 stated that ragweed would "stimulate the gastric flow not only through the liver and gall duct. . .[but would] cleanse those areas about the caecum and appendix."

And for those susceptible to hay fever, who suffer throughout the pollen-bearing season, the readings claimed that ragweed could help reduce this oversensitivity:

Now, as we find, there are conditions which tend to disturb the body at specific periods. Hence, as is indicated, there are certain seasons or periods when the vibrations of the body, or the relationships which are established in the nerve centers, are such as to cause the body to become allergic to conditions which exist in or under certain environs, or certain pressure experienced by climatic reactions in the body.

These reactions come from what may be called or set up as

vibrations in certain centers between sympathetic and cerebrospinal system, and thus the body in such periods is subject to conditions which manifest in irritation to mucous membranes of the nasal passage and throat, bronchi and larynx, or, as sometimes called, rose fever or such natures. These, for this body, are particularly from the ragweed.

Thus, we would find in this particular season, before there is the blossoming of same, the body should take quantities of this weed. Brew same, prepare, take internally and thus war or ward against the activity of this upon the body itself.

Then, through the period, also take that [inhalant] as an antiseptic reaction upon the nerves of the nasal passages, or the olfactory nerves of the body.

These will prevent, then, the recurrent conditions which have been and are a part of the experience of the body. This will enable the body to become immune because of the very action of this weed upon the digestive system, and the manner it will act with the assimilating body, too. Well, just don't get too heavy, for it will make for an increase in the amount of assimilation and distribution of food values for the body.

Thus we would prepare the compound in this manner: Take a pint cup, gather the tender leaves of the weed, don't cram in but just fill level. Put this in an enamel or a glass container and then the same amount...of distilled water, see? Reduce this to half the quantity by very slow boiling, not hard but slow boiling, strain and add sufficient grain alcohol as a preservative.

Begin and take it through the fifteen days of July and the whole of August, daily, half a teaspoonful each day.

Thus, we will find better eliminations, we will find better assimilation, we will find better distribution of the activities of foods in the body.

5347-1

See the CF on Liver: Torpid and other pertinent Files.

It is recommended that you consult a physician before using this product.

RAY'S OINTMENT AND RAY'S SOLUTION

Ray's products were formulated by a Roanoke chemist, Thomas Ray Wirsing, who later became involved in preparing medicines for individuals who had received the formulas in their Cayce readings. His medicated products for treatment of various skin irritations were recommended in about 15 readings. Most of these were for cases of eczema and athlete's foot, as well as dermatitis and poison ivy. Use of the ointment was advised in the majority of these cases, while the liquid (solution) was indicated in cases of poison ivy and in one case of athlete's foot.

Regarding application of these compounds for athlete's foot, this reading comments:

...feet, ankles, these we would bathe in Ray's Ointment and we would relieve the tendencies for infectious forces produced by this acidity in the system. 5261-1

A report following the above reading stated that after application of the ointment, symptoms of athlete's foot disappeared.

Q-5. Please suggest a remedy for heat rash and athlete's foot.
A-5. As indicated, the vitamin forces will be well for those internal troubles, see. Ray's Ointment or Ray's Solution as prepared for athlete's foot is in accordance with the best conditions, as we find. This applied also to the rash will be most beneficial. 361-15

Q-4. To cure athlete's foot?
A-4. As we find, the best that may be had of this nature is that we have indicated oft—the preparation made by those in the vicinity of Roanoke, Virginia. 984-5

Make local application to the eruptions and the broken tissue with Ray's eczema ointment. This carries these properties that will allay. 477-2

For an individual with dermatitis, one reading advised:

Obtain and apply Ray's Ointment for the rash. We find that this will relieve these tensions and alleviate disturbances. 3620-1

And for eczema:

Bathe off the affected parts each day, at least once a day, using Cuticura soap, and then apply Ray's prescription for eczema. The character or nature of the properties here will allay, but of course will not be curative forces. They are merely to allay the irritation. 2518-1

Then when there is a rash—or the irritation, apply Ray's Ointment. The salicylic activities here will allay the irritation, and—with the osteopathic corrections *and* the properties taken internally—will aid the system. 3109-1

For more information, consult the CFs on Acne, Athlete's Foot, Dermatitis, Eczema, and Poison Ivy.

SAFFRON

Yellow or American Saffron is an herb sometimes used as a natural dye, and known primarily for its diaphoretic, or perspiration-inducing qualities. It was recommended approximately 190 times in the readings for its beneficial effects on digestion, in cases such as psoriasis, toxemia, stomach ulcers and incoordination between assimilations and eliminations.

These properties [saffron in water] as a tonic or stimulant in the assimilating system would produce and keep, with the digestive forces, the proper reactions as to prevent recurrence of disturbing conditions that have been indicated for this body heretofore. 556-16

The reading quoted above also noted that the taking of the saffron tea would prevent foods from causing flatulence (gas):

The saffron will assimilate and coordinate with the gastric juices of the *digestive* system, in such a way and manner as to eliminate that character of poisons that saps the vitality of the muco-membranes of the digestive and intestinal system. 4510-1

[Saffron tea] stimulates better strength through the activities of the lymph and emunctory circulation in the alimentary canal. 257-215

The saffron [should be taken] once or twice each day, that the irritation [of ulcers] may be kept down and *preventing* any reoccurrence. 348-5

This should be kept up not in a haphazard manner, but until there is a better condition physically created throughout the alimentary canal. Take it for two, three, four, five days, a week, ten days—leave it off [for] a few days, and then have it prepared again and take again. 257-215

The following directions for preparation of the tea are typical:

The saffron tea—teaspoonful to a pint [or about a pinch to a teacup], and this allowed to simmer as making tea, or just brew as tea. This, of course, may be made a pint at a time, but of course not a whole pint taken at once. . .   1419-3

Or, boiling water may be poured over a pinch of the herb in a teacup, allowing it to steep 15 minutes before straining and drinking.

Reading 257-14 stated that the saffron tea should be made fresh every two days.

Some readings advised taking the saffron tea about half an hour before each meal to prepare the system for better assimilations. Reading 5545-1 stated that this would coat the stomach and thus aid digestion.

Frequently a tea made from slippery elm bark was to be taken during the same period as the saffron. Some readings advised taking one or the other, a few said to combine the two, while others advised that they be alternated daily.

For more information, consult the CFs on Stomach: Indigestion and Gastritis; Stomach: Ulcers; and Skin: Psoriasis.

SCAR FORMULA [2015-10]

The Cayce formula now most commonly used for scars was given in only one reading, although in most of the 16 readings on scars, variations of this formula were suggested.

The "classic" combination, from reading 2015-10, has been used successfully in the removal of severe burn scars, and even in treatment of the burns themselves, and consists of camphorated olive oil, lanolin and peanut oil.

For more information consult the CF on Skin: Scars.

SEA SALT AND KELP SALT

Kelp salt was mentioned about 30 times in the Cayce readings. Many of these readings also mention that if preferred, "deep sea salt" may be substituted. Both are high in natural trace minerals, especially iodine. Kelp is a product derived from seaweed. Sea salt refers to salt extracted directly from sea water rather than mined from deposits found on land.

The sea salt should be preferably used from the kelp rather than that from sea water. Kelp, to be sure, is a plant that

carries all the properties of same; and this taken as seasoning for corn bread or seasoning of certain characters of vegetables *after* they are prepared is good in the diet.   658-15

. . .*especially* use as the seasoning the kelp or sea salt as is from kelp—this will add to the vibrations of the body.1247-1

Kelp salt and sea salt were recommended not only for general use but also in a variety of cases involving a lack of sufficient iodine in the system. In cases of arthritis particularly, this dietary method of adding iodine to the system was suggested:

In the diet, through this activity, keep away from salt. Only use either deep sea salt or kelp salt. This we would use regularly.   4049-1

Kelp salt was also recommended in one commonly followed reading for baldness in which dietary instructions stressed iodine-containing foods.

SKIN FRESHENER [404-8]

For a woman who asked for a good skin freshener, the readings suggested mixing ½ pint of olive oil with 1 ounce of rosewater, a few drops of glycerine and 1 ounce of a 10% solution of alcohol, and shake these well together. This is a skin invigorator.
    See the CF on Skin: Complexion: Cosmetics; also see in Dr. Reilly's book "Beauty Problems."

SPIRITS OF CAMPHOR

Camphor is used medically as an irritant and stimulant, and spirits of camphor is made by combining camphor with alcohol. This substance was mentioned in about 235 readings, and is probably best known as an ingredient in the Colds Liniment, in combination with equal parts of mutton tallow and spirits of turpentine. The camphor plays its part by "assisting in penetration *and* in healing. . ." (2509-1) In addition, however, spirits of camphor was recommended in other types of massage formulas, in combination with such ingredients as sassafras oil, cedar wood oil, Nujol, witch hazel and olive oil. (See in Dr. Reilly's book "Cayce Massage Mixtures.")

100

Spirits of camphor is also recommended as an application for the feet, particularly in cases of bunions, callouses, corns and ingrown toenails:

These [ingrown toenails] as we find would respond to the dampening of baking soda with spirits of camphor and putting a small quantity of same on cotton, or alone, under the tip of the nail, close to the irritated place. This will remove the condition, if used daily—or nightly.   1770-4

This will tend to make the nails crumble at once or within the month; but then the new nails should come in normally, provided the other applications are kept up as indicated, and the changes wrought in the glandular activity by the diets outlined for the body.   2315-1

For corns:

Bathe the limb from [the] knee down with warm olive oil. Then apply the saturated solution of spirits of camphor, with bicarbonate of soda. Even spread it on, as a very thin layer, see? bandaging this with a *thin* cloth...about the limb and foot. Let this remain over the evening, or night...We find this will bring the better condition, better circulation, remove the callouses, and give ease.   3776-13

Spirits of camphor may also be used to treat sunburn:

As for the acute conditions—we would daub or apply spirits of camphor, by using tufts of cotton. Then in an hour or two hours afterward have a tepid bath, and then apply peanut oil.
303-33

For more information, consult the CFs on Colds; Burns: Sunburn; and Feet: Weakness, Swelling, etc.

SULPHUR LAXATIVE COMPOUND [5016-1]

The Sulphur Laxative Compound is a formula containing equal parts of sulphur, cream of tartar and Rochelle salts, that was recommended in about 40 readings. They frequently stressed that this mixture be stirred *thoroughly* and often suggested the use of a mortar and pestle for this purpose. Sometimes Epsom salts was indicated instead of Rochelle salts. If following a particular reading which differs from above formula, one should have the ingredients prepared (mixed thoroughly) by a pharmacist. *In either case it should be done only by or on the prescription of a physician.*

The mixture acts as a mild laxative and blood purifier (according to the readings) and was, therefore, indicated to stimulate and coordinate the eliminating functions. It was frequently mentioned in cases of boils and carbuncles, eczema, acne, psoriasis, dermatitis, and for general purification and cleansing of the system:

This would be taken as a cleanser for the whole system.
1711-1

As a laxative it is better than many because it is mild and not habit-forming:

It is well to use same. It is not habit-forming, it will not injure the intestinal tract nor cause any great disturbance—if there is the minimal activity of the body.
2843-4

An individual with poor circulation, obesity, psoriasis and cysts was advised that "These properties. . .will so purify the system that cold and congestion, the cough, the shortness of breath, will be *greatly* benefited." (2455-1)

Dosage of the Sulphur Laxative varies in recommendation from one-fourth of a teaspoon to one teaspoon a day, though the usual daily dosage recommended was one level teaspoon. This should be taken in the morning, before meals. Some readings state that it may be taken either dry or in water, while others specify warm or hot water:

The dose would be a level teaspoonful of the mixture each day, stirred in a glass of water—preferably *hot* water, so that the assimilations of this will make for the activity through the system.
357-5

Most readings state that the Sulphur Laxative Compound should be taken daily, until the original amount (usually three tablespoonsful) mixed together has been exhausted. This would take about nine days in the average recommendation.

The main precaution to observe when taking the Sulphur Laxative is to avoid getting the feet wet, since at this time the system will be more susceptible to colds:

As we find, these properties which we will indicate are the better to purify the system, provided the taking of same is in keeping with the activities of the body and the body doesn't get

the feet wet or damp during the periods that these would be taken. For, if they did, it might rebound or cause more ill disturbance than help!

This doesn't mean that you can't take a bath during the time, but you musn't get out in the snow or rain or wet, or to have the body damp from the rain or the like! For this will tend to open the pores, the taking of these properties, and is effective upon the whole of the circulation, purifying and coordinating the whole of the circulation through [the] alimentary canal, the activity of the liver, the respiratory system, and the flow and activity of the kidneys.

These should purify the body.   2462-3

Also one was advised against wearing shoes "with the feet wet, for it would cause disturbance in other portions of the body." (3678-1)

Mrs. [2455] was also told not to spend too much time in a standing position:

. . .do not get them [the feet] wet as from outdoor activity, or housework. Do not allow the body to become too tired from standing on the feet too long. For, these would tend to aggravate rather than to aid in better eliminations. For, under the wet conditions, the body would be more easily susceptible to cold.   2455-1

Dietary precautions sometimes accompanied the recommendations. Reading 2462-3 states: "*Do not* eat excesses of starch or fats during these periods. . ."

We would have those foods that will make for body building, with not too great an amount of weight but those that tend—as it were—to make for a laxative reaction for the body; as citrus fruit juices, raw fresh vegetables, any of the cereals (though these should not be taken on the same day, or at the same meal at least, with the citrus fruit juices); whole wheat as a mush, and things of such natures would be more preferable for the body during the four days the above mixture is being taken.   357-5

Then drink plenty of water through the day, at least six to eight tumblers [glasses] full.   2341-1

Case [2803] was advised to avoid eating fish and shellfish during the period that Sulphur Laxative was being taken, and [3261] and [2674] were told to eat very little meat. In a few readings the apple diet, which also aids in cleansing the system, was advised.

Also recommended occasionally along with the Sulphur Laxative were products such as Atomidine* and Castoria.

One person, [1711], was told to take this compound three to four days, leave off a day, and:

> ...*then* take *one* minim [drop] of Atomidine* in half a glass of water before the morning meal each day for three or four days. Then leave this off for a day. Then begin with taking the combination or compound as indicated for three to four more days. Then this may be left off for several days—three, four to five.
>
> Then begin all over again; and keep these up from time to time until the system has purified itself.   1711-1

> After these properties [Sulphur Laxative] have been taken and have acted upon the system. . .we find it would be well to take a full day of the Fletcher's Castoria. This would be taken half a teaspoonful every hour until there is the absorption in the system *and* the elimination or activity from same. 357-5

> As we find, it would be well to first cleanse the system of the effects of those properties which have been indicated—that is, the sulphur and the other properties, by the use of Castoria *and* the alkalizer that has been indicated (the Magnesia) continued for at least two or three days.   1208-16

For more information, consult the CFs on Skin: Acne; Eczema; Psoriasis; Dermatitis; Boils; and Carbuncles.

A notation from Gladys Davis: Remember, the above quoted cases are of different ages and with specific problems; the advice as to combinations of treatments, medicines, dosages, etc., would not apply generally. The last case quoted above, [1208], was a small child. Study the pertinent CF with your Cooperating Physician to decide whether or not any of the advice is proper for you.

It is recommended that you consult a physician before using this product.

SWEET SPIRITS OF NITRE

Sweet spirits of nitre was recommended in about 50 readings, primarily as a cleanser and stimulus to the kidneys and bladder. In some cases it was to be taken in combination with

---

*It is recommended that you consult a physician before using this product.

other properties, such as oil of juniper, to act on the gall duct. Sweet spirits of nitre was recently discontinued by its U.S. manufacturers. A possible substitute, also recommended for the kidneys, is watermelon seed tea.

SYRUP OF FIGS

A laxative preparation known as Syrup of Figs was recommended in over 90 readings. It contained extract of figs and, according to the readings, had a senna base. Because of its gentleness, this preparation was a preferred choice in many cases where the eliminations needed stimulating. It was also regarded as a stimulus to the assimilations, which would "act with the gastric juices of the system and. . .increase the flow through the alimentary canal." (378-7)

In many cases, Syrup of Figs was mentioned along with other laxatives, all of which were considered good options. It was often to be alternated with either other senna-based laxatives such as Castoria or with mineral-based laxatives or both.

Some readings specified a particular brand of the figs syrup, such as Caldwell's or California, but many others did not. This product is presumably no longer on the market, although a possibly related product, Dr. Caldwell's Laxative (made by Glenbrook Labs), is currently available.

SYRUP OF SQUILL

Syrup of Squill was recommended in about 50 readings, predominately in cases of cold and congestion, pneumonia and poor eliminations. Squill refers to a bulb related to the onion. It has been used as a nauseant and expectorant, and its action and uses are similar to those of digitalis. The readings variously suggested its use as an aid to the respiratory system, as a decongestant, and occasionally as a cardiac (heart stimulant). This preparation was claimed to be more beneficial for babies and children than for adults because it interacted best with the developmental processes of a growing body. An average dosage was five to ten drops every two to four hours. Syrup of Squill is a prescription item available at some pharmacies.

TIM [1800-20]

Tim is a compound recommended in about 60 readings, primarily in cases of hemorrhoids, but also in a few instances of skin irritation, including pruritus, eczema, abrasions and boils. The formulas given vary somewhat from reading to reading, but the Tim formula in general use at present contains iodine and benzoin in a natural ointment base. Instructions for use are as follows:

The directions would be to apply as an ointment to affected portions once or twice each day. Rest as much as possible *after* application, with the feet elevated *above* the head. It'll cure it!
1800-20

Hemorrhoids is a condition involving enlarged and varicose veins in the lower portion of the rectum and the tissues about the anus. Apparently Tim acts not only as a palliative measure to reduce the inflammation and pain, but also aids in restoring normal conditions. Additional comments are found in the readings:

For an antiseptic and to reduce the tendencies of plethora [excess of blood] in those portions that cause distress, use the ointment known as Tim. This will act with the manipulative forces to not only reduce the swelling and the painfulness, but to produce or cause coagulation such as to do away with those protuberances which make for the distress.
Following each stool the Tim ointment should be used, or after the body is ready for retiring. This will be found to be more effective than any other application.   4873-1

Consistently used, it will not only remove the cause but remove the hemorrhoids.   257-200

This applied, with the proper manipulation in the lumbar and sacral region, will *permanently* relieve this body of such conditions.   654-3

Tim may be applied whenever necessary for rapid relief:

That as being applied [Tim] will relieve in at least three to four applications, using each time when these show projections, or when stools are taken.   147-34

Occasionally Tim was suggested following enemas and colonics:

. . .the general reaction and the use of Tim after such an activity [colonic] would be most advisable and advantageous.
257-208

In cases of hemorrhoids requiring internal application, use of a bulb syringe such as an ear syringe was advised, and the Tim may be heated to make it more easily injectable:

Then if it is of the protruding type, of course the local application. If the internal type, or the blind type, of course the injection. . .
257-210

. . .this would be well to be injected, in a small syringe, or in a manner that same may reach the upper valve or portion of the system that irritation is produced in. Using a small amount of same as an ointment of evenings, only when the body rests, on and about that portion where the trouble exists.
5566-5

In some instances both external and internal application was advised:

After each stool, and there is the cleansing, then use Tim as an ointment *and* an injection. This having an astringent and a curative and an allaying reaction to the inflammatory conditions will, with the exercise, with the food for the intestinal system, tend to eliminate entirely the disturbance.
257-172

For more information, consult the CF on Hemorrhoids.

Gladys Davis added this information: In some cases other preparations—then on the market—were recommended for hemorrhoids (such as Pazo's Ointment). This was true in my own case, as I was allergic to the snuff, or tobacco, one of the main ingredients. The name Tim was given in the readings themselves after our good friend, Mr. [195], whose nickname was Tim, prepared the formula indicated in his own reading and, getting good results, continued to make it in those early days for others who had it advised in their readings.

TONICINE

This product was popular during the 1930s, sold as a "gonadal tonic" by Reed and Carnrick on a prescription basis. The ingredients are not known, though one reading said that it was made from glandular secretions or glandular reactions.

Tonicine was recommended in about 60 readings, primarily for glandular imbalances and for conditions of the generative organs such as menopause and pelvic disorders. Formula from 636-1,* a glandular tonic, is a possible substitute.

TORIS COMPOUND

Toris Compound was a laxative preparation recommended about 70 times in the readings primarily for inadequate eliminations and toxemia. This preparation was found to be beneficial because it stimulated the excretory system without irritation to tissue or to the lymph circulation. Ragweed Laxative [369-12]* is a possible substitute.

VALENTINE'S LIVER EXTRACT

Valentine's Liver Extract is a liquid extract of edible mammalian liver, approved by the medical profession since 1929 for treatment of pernicious anemia and related deficiency diseases. It is especially valued for its supply of B vitamins. A modified version of this product, Valentine's Liver Extract with Iron, is indicated in treatment of secondary anemias due to iron deficiencies. Valentine's Liver Extract—in most cases, the plain version—was recommended in about 15 readings. The Cayce source said it was a blood and body builder, and recommended it primarily in cases of anemia and general debilitation.

During the periods of rest from the taking of the Atomidine,* we would would take enzymes that will act upon the body in creating for a digestive force, and the active elements that are lacking in creating the balance through the system. As we find, these may be combined for this body in *two* elements; Valentine's Extract of Liver *and* Ventriculin with Iron.

1173-1

As a tonic we would take Valentine's juices of liver, as an extract, for its activity. Occasionally we would combine with same the White's Codliver Oil Tablets; these would be taken one every third day.

1179-1

Valentine's Liver Extract may be taken in preference to the liver itself if it is so desired, but this when taken should be in

*It is recommended that you consult a physician before using this product.

small doses and taken for two or three days at a time, then leave it off for two or three days and begin again.   856-1

VEGETABLE JUICER

Fresh raw vegetables and their juices were recommended in many Cayce readings, and about twenty advised the use of a juicer to extract these valuable juices:

At least once each day take an ounce of raw carrot juice. Use a juicer to extract the juice from fresh raw carrots.   243-33

Once or twice a week take vegetable juices that would be prepared by using a vegetable juicer, but only using the vegetables for same that would combine well.   1968-3

The juices from these are to be prepared fresh each day.
462-13

...each day have at least an ounce of vegetable juices; such as a combination of lettuce and carrots especially, and at times including celery juice—to strengthen the general nerve forces of the body. These would be the raw juices, of course.2154-2

Take an ounce of carrot juice *each day*. Use a juice extractor to obtain the juice from fresh, raw carrots. Take this each day for at least a month, then leave off for a week; then begin all over again...these are for the better eliminations, you see. Especially the carrot juice, in combination with the rest of the diet, is to aid in dissolving the poisons and eliminating them.
2180-1

But the beet juice should be extracted, or prepared as in a juicer ...But the pure juice is needed, not only the salts but those elements that are within, which will tend to alleviate these pressures and tendencies.   2946-1

The above reading implies that the fresh juices contain more valuable nutrients than could be obtained by substituting the canned variety. Because these nutrients are quickly lost in storage, the juice should be made fresh daily.

The varieties of vegetable juices most often mentioned were beet, carrot, celery, lettuce, spinach and tomato. Beet juice was specified in some cases involving arthritis, neuritis, and muscular disease, and carrot juice for arthritis and the eyes.

VENTRICULIN

Ventriculin and Ventriculin with Iron were manufactured by Parke-Davis and Company until the mid or late 1950s. Ventriculin was a substance derived from the gastric tissue of hogs, in a powder form that was taken orally. Ventriculin was used to stimulate the formation of reticulocytes (a type of red blood cell) and was recommended by the manufacturer as a specific for pernicious anemia. Ventriculin was recommended in about 55 readings and Ventriculin with Iron in about 40. The readings suggested Ventriculin primarily in cases of anemia but also for general debilitation, poor assimilations, and a wide range of other conditions, including scleroderma as an extreme example. It may be that the Cayce source saw this substance as a stimulus to the assimilations and thus also to the formation of more red blood cells. The doctor's commentary in the Scleroderma CF lists and compares the following possible substitutes for Ventriculin: Converzyme, Digestant, and Entozyme. All of these are prescription items.

VIOLET RAY

The Violet Ray, as it was called in the Cayce readings, is basically a high voltage, low amperage source of static electricity. Today it is usually referred to as a high frequency device. The name Violet Ray is derived from the color of the electrical discharge and should not be confused with ultraviolet light. In the first three decades of the 1900s, the Violet Ray was widely distributed and used in a large variety of medical conditions.

This device consists of a base, which is held in the hand, and into which can be inserted the various types of glass applicators available, such as the bulb, double-eye, comb-rake and rod, with shape depending on the manner of usage intended. Some of the applicators recommended in the readings, such as the rectal and vaginal attachments, are no longer made today. Therefore, categories such as hemorrhoids and pelvic disorders, in which these obsolete applicators were suggested, will not be discussed here.

This appliance was mentioned in the readings approximately 825 times. The cases in which the Violet Ray was given as a part of treatment are many and varied, and its use in only the major categories will be included here, in approximate order of frequency with which they were mentioned.

Circulation:

The primary function of the Violet Ray is to stimulate the superficial circulation. In the process, additional beneficial effects can be achieved:

This would be to create a balance of circulation through the superficial portion of the body, causing a bettering of the conditions. 436-4

This will make for the abilities of the body to rest better. It will tend to make for strengthening of the body, by the toning of the circulation—as combined with the adjustments that are taken. 1611-2

The body should use the Violet Ray over the whole circulatory system, for five to ten minutes, to stimulate the circulation and the nerve centers, sufficiently to start the proper elimination. Do that and we will be able to reduce the condition in the throat and over the system by absorption.
4831-2

The readings stated that osteopathic adjustments would improve the condition of [679]:

. . .as also would the stimulating of the ganglia that are relieved by having the pressures in the [spinal] segments relieved or released, see? through the addition of the electrical vibrations from the plain Violet Ray over segments that are changed, which would bring the superficial circulation to such an activity as to cause the flow of the blood supply through same. Thus not only would the distresses in those particular portions be relieved, but the impulse for the circulation through the head and the neck and to the optic forces and to all portions of the face would be such as to *improve* the functioning of the organs; bringing a nearer normal condition.
679-2

Nerves:

If this is taken just before retiring it should aid in the ability to rest, and [in] quieting the nerves. 540-12

This treatment is to so charge the centers of the nervous system as to make for (with the changes created in the activities of that assimilated, in its distribution through the system) better coordination *between* the sympathetic and cerebrospinal nervous system. It would produce stimuli to the *ganglia* in the cerebrospinal and sympathetic coordinating centers.   259-7

...this [condition] is the incoordination between *impulse* and the reactions from the cerebrospinal and sympathetic nerve system. The osteopathic adjustments, and especially the heat from the high vibrations of the Violet Ray in the manner indicated, will aid.   1540-3

...apply to the body the correct vibrations [from the Violet Ray] that will give the incentives to the nerve centers to become rejuvenated again...   269-1

Spinal Subluxations:
   A subluxation is a partial dislocation or sprain. To relieve resultant pressures, use of the Violet Ray both alone and in conjunction with osteopathic adjustments was often advised. It is probably best not to use the Violet Ray on the same days the adjustments are given, as in reading 1584-1, which recommends applying the Violet Ray "when the adjustments are *not* being taken!"

   This [Violet Ray treatment] may be taken at the same periods when the preventative measures are taken for the strengthening of the muscular forces in the lower portion of the body, by the gentle massage...   772-3

...and the period of treatment would last for the length of time *necessary* to *bring* relaxation to the system, whether two minutes or fifteen minutes!   1315-1

Eyes:
   The Violet Ray was recommended in cases of cataracts, blindness and myopia, among others. Generally, the double-eye applicator (some readings simply stated "eye applicator") was suggested for use in these instances, although sometimes application in the head and neck regions with the bulb attachment was preferred. It is stressed that the double-eye applicator should always be used with the eyes closed.

   With the application of the violet applicator to the eye proper, we will find that there will be more response from the optic centers proper, and the relief gradually through the stimulating of the circulation to remove those pressures *on* same as cause...the neuralgia-like condition as exists there. The condition in same...[is] produced by pressure on [the] optic nerve back of [the] eye proper, from sedimentation in [the] system and lack of coordination in the eliminations, first producing neuritis in the general system, settling—from strain on [the] eye. . .[This condition should be treated by the Violet Ray, or] direct rays of the character of lights.   2-19

Q-2. Left eye feels strained. What do you find and what suggestion?
A-2. Only pressures in the nerve system and thus the vibrations from the Violet Ray for five to ten minutes each evening, of course along the upper dorsal and the back portion along the cervical would be better and across the head and over the eye. These would be relaxing to same.   261-24

Anemia:

To bring at the present time the better conditions to the body we would use those of the manipulation as applied by the hands rather than the vibratory forces, still using the electrical forces as would be applied from the Violet Ray, that we may bring more of the blood supply through the nerve reaction in and through the tissue in [the] exterior portion, as well as through the deeper tissue. Apply across the abdomen very thoroughly, that we may awaken the functioning of the liver, spleen, and those portions in the digestive tract. 979-3

Arthritis:
In cases of arthritis the taking of gold* and soda prior to Violet Ray applications was often recommended. The readings explained that this combination would aid in "Assisting the eliminations, aiding the system to function through the glands—where assimilation has been hindered, that causes tautness in the centers about nerve ends, where they join in the joints or sinews of the body. "Do not apply the Ray of such a period as to produce irritation, but of sufficient that there may be a stimulated lymphatic and capillary circulation." (120-2)

And the activities of the Violet Ray are only to make for the electrical rejuvenation of nerve energies that have been depleted through the inactivity of the whole system of the body.   676-1

The Violet Ray is recommended "to overcome these tendencies or to relieve these pressures in the bursae along the joints, along the nerves of the tendons and leaders—superficial activity, to be sure." (888-1)

---

*It is recommended that you consult a physician before using this product.

General Debilitation:

This will give the "pick up" or the stimulation that is needed for what might be called the recharging of the centers along the cerebrospinal system, so that there is better coordination between the ganglia of the cerebrospinal and the sympathetic nerve system.   1196-17

To do this will prevent the central nervous system batteries from running down.
It'll pick the body up!   2528-4

Eliminations:

We would use the hand Violet Ray; this for the nerve forces will aid especially, if it is *gradually* used across the abdominal area; this given just before the body retires, or when it is prepared for rest of evenings, will aid in better rest and will aid in relaxing the body and stimulating better eliminations.
                                                                         1553-20

Baldness and Falling Hair:

The Violet Ray provides "A stimulation to any portion of the body for greater activity, [and] by not too much but as using the comb of such a hand Violet Ray machine through the hair and head, will make for such stimulation as to make more growth of the hair and also a better growth of the hair." (1120-2)

In reading 5339-1, use of the Violet Ray was to be alternated with cycles of taking Atomidine.*

Glands:

This [Violet Ray] is a high voltage, stimulating all centers [glands] that are as the crossroads, the connections between the various portions of the physical-body functioning, the mental attitudes and attainments, as well as the sources of [spiritual] supply; which [influences] arose by the choice of the entity in entering this particular temple, this individual temple [body].   263-13

The readings on goitre relate closely to this subject of glands, particularly the thyroid gland. In such cases, Atomidine* was frequently a part of the treatment recommended, although it was not to be taken on the same days as the Violet Ray treatment.

---

*It is recommended that you consult a physician before using this product.

We would have each day the Violet Ray treatment, along the spine and over the throat where there are those tendencies for the non-activity of the glands from the thyroids and those accumulations and the fullness that appears in the throat. These will naturally be somewhat irritated at times by the electrical vibrations, but with the taking of properties for the glands themselves [Atomidine*] the body will gradually adjust itself. These [applications] will make for better conditions and *electrify*, as it were, the energies of the system. 421-10

As indicated, the application of the Violet Ray over this portion [throat] of the system will tend to make for better coordination in the circulation, both superficial and internal, as there is the stimulation to the circulation; and, as we find, this should overcome the tendencies for disturbance in the vocal box. 270-32

Q-1. Does the body have goitre?
A-1. It is the condition we are giving here for the Violet Ray, in the thyroid region. This is enlarged gland as yet, but may turn into such [goitre] if the system is allowed to secrete those particles that will draw and settle in this portion of the body. 2790-3

A report following this reading stated that the Violet Ray was used regularly, the swelling subsided, and no goitre developed.

Neurasthenia:
Neurasthenia in its various forms generally involves tiring easily, lack of energy, various aches and pains, and disinclination to activity.

[Apply]. . .the vibrations of the plain or regular Violet Ray. This will aid in *equalizing* with the rest of that applied the general circulation and nerve distribution.
With these corrections, and especially with the vibrations of the Violet Ray applied in the manner given, these will create more activity through the eliminating *systems,* and *especially* through the alimentary canal. 5640-1

Possession:
The Violet Ray was recommended almost invariably in such cases:

---

*It is recommended that you consult a physician before using this product.

These treatments will tend to make for the raising of the vibrations of the body, disassociating the effects of repressions in the system, producing better coordination throughout.   1572-1

This may cause illness or nausea for the first one or two times. If it does, leave it off for a day or two or give it for a shorter period of time. But if these vibrations are used, there will be less opportunity for the attacks that cause such hallucinations.   3158-2

When aroused from this subjection of the subconscious to control, by the performing of such impressions, use the low electrical forces to change vibrations through the body. The hand machine Violet Ray should be sufficient. . .Not too long a period, just sufficient to disassociate the flexures as would nominally come as there is the regaining of the *normal* reactions of the body.   3075-1

Precautions Advised:

The use of the Violet Ray is, according to the readings, incompatible with certain other treatments, or substances that may be taken internally. For instance, the Violet Ray should not be applied any time Atomidine* is being taken, although the two may be alternated according to whatever cycle is established, allowing a rest period of two or three days between the time one is left off and the other begun. This includes other medicines and drugs as well:

Do not take medicinal properties while these [vibrations] *are being applied, see?* either the osteopathic forces or the electrical treatments! Take no drugs.   4843-1

X-rays should not be taken during periods when the Violet Ray is in use:

As indicated, if the X-ray flashes are used we would not use the Violet Ray, especially when they are given every day! We have given this again and again!

The hand massage, as indicated, would be well—gently—to induce sleep, in the evenings. But leave off the machine while the X-ray treatments are being given!   325-64

Alcohol should also be avoided, even in the form of fumes as are inhaled through the charred oak keg*:

---

*It is recommended that you consult a physician before using this product.

This [Violet Ray treatment] strengthens any vibration and is good for the nerve system, when alcohols in no form are taken.

538-3

. . .do not use electrical forces or treatments when there is inhalation of alcoholic forces in the body. This burns, or retards, or irritates rather than assists.   4253-1

Abstain from *any* intoxicating drinks of *any* kind! This means even beer too! Too much of these, with the electrical forces (if they are to be taken), will be *detrimental* to the better conditions of the body.

Electricity and alcohol don't work together! It burns tissue, and is not good for *anybody!*   323-1

One reading warns against combining the use of the Violet Ray with yoga exercises:

Q-2. Is the yoga practice of Kriya causing any ill effects?
A-2. As indicated, this is very well to continue with these treatments; for these exercises have a stimulating effect. However, *do not* use these during the period the Violet Ray is used, for that week!   813-2

Duration of time advised for individual Violet Ray applications varied widely from reading to reading. In the following reading, [1861] was told that one and a half minutes was plenty:

As to the Violet Ray application—there has been indicated a specific time. This has been overstepped at times, with the idea that if a little would do good more would do more good; while at times more does harm rather than good! It is as an overtaxation even to a strong muscular force may weaken, may even deter the best activity. Do not overstrain, but keep the Violet Ray—and not more than the minute or minute and a half.   1861-11

Apply it in such a manner as to expect and to obtain the revivifying of the body-forces themselves.   3060-1

For more details and related treatments, consult the appropriate CFs.

It is recommended that you consult a physician before using this product.

WATERMELON SEED TEA

Watermelon seed tea is a diuretic recommended in the readings about 75 times, particularly as a stimulant to the functioning of the kidneys and bladder.

This will clarify those conditions that cause reactions in the kidneys and bladder, for, the lack of eliminations and the slowing up of the circulation causes a greater quantity of drosses to be held in the system, and these need to be eliminated from the body.

More will be eliminated through using this stimuli for the kidney activity than in most any way.   1695-2

[Take watermelon seed tea] to reduce this activity through the kidneys' affectations, and to alleviate the quantities of water that accumulate through the abdominal area.

These, as we find in the present, will keep the eliminations in such manners that we will bring the conditions that may *eliminate* these disturbances from this body.   1148-1

We would use occasionally the watermelon seed tea, which will materially aid in eliminating this from the system. There is just sufficient of the nitre here, and in the right proportions, to act upon the gastric flow to remove these disturbances which cause the pressures.

...This, after being taken for two or three days, should make for such changes in the activity of the coordination of the eliminations of the system as to relieve the disturbances entirely...The use of the character of nitre as combined in the watermelon seed tea will *not* cause a disturbance in the system.   470-28

There is sufficient of the nitre and other properties in this that if drunk it will be beneficial to clearing up the inflammation through the areas not only of the kidneys and bladder but will also aid in the ovarian disturbance. 2048-8

The delivery [of baby] should be normal, as we find, but there will be trouble with the kidneys unless proper precautions are taken to keep the activities well. Hence very small quantities of watermelon seed tea would be well, soon after the birth of the babe.   951-7

Watermelon seed tea should be made in the proportion of about one teaspoon to a pint (or about a pinch to a teacup) of boiling water, steeped for about 15 minutes, and taken once a week or oftener. Some readings advised that it was best taken in small quantities several times a day rather than a larger amount taken once a day. The tea should be made fresh every few days:

...do not keep longer, even in the ice box, than two or three days; for this becomes then retroactive, of course, by the action of air and of properties that would be in the same location throwing off their emanations. It is better that it be put in a bottle and corked, even in the ice box—when kept at all; but warmed to be taken.   569-25

For more information, consult the CFs on Kidneys, and Bladder: Cystitis.

WET CELL APPLIANCE

The Wet Cell Appliance was referred to by the readings about 975 times, *in all cases indicated for specific conditions rather than general use.* It was suggested in a wide variety of physical and mental disturbances, such as nerves and incoordination of nervous systems, abnormal children, multiple sclerosis, insanity, arthritis, paralysis, Parkinson's disease, and deafness, and seems to be most often indicated in those cases requiring rebuilding of tissue and restoration of bodily functions.

The Wet Cell is a battery, producing a very small but measurable electric current. This current is of the frequency and type that supposedly stimulates the growth of nerve tissue, and strengthens the connections between nerve tissue. Attachments are made from the battery, using lead wires, to specific areas of the body, which vary according to the condition diagnosed. Almost always specific solutions were to be included in the circuit, to supply certain elements to the body vibratorially. Those solutions most commonly recommended were spirits of camphor, gold chloride,* silver nitrate, and Atomidine.* The readings stated that in some cases this would be more beneficial than taking certain minerals internally, such as gold and iodine.

We find that any of such solutions may be given to the body, as we have indicated, through this manner; causing the activity of same without it passing through the system itself,

---

*It is recommended that you consult a physician before using this product.

for it may be directed to various organs of the system that are in need of such elements as to the glands in any portion of the system that receive impulse from the cerebrospinal system, or from the sympathetic or the vegetative system, or from any of the ganglia of the *lymph* or *emunctory* circulation that forms itself in portions of the body.   1800-25

For more information, consult the booklet on the electrical appliances described in the Edgar Cayce readings and the appropriate CFs.

It is recommended that you consult a physician before using this product.

WHEAT GERM OIL

Wheat germ oil as a dietary supplement was suggested in about 25 readings, particularly for its vitamin E content. It was especially recommended for arthritis and for physical adjustments involving the generative organs, as in the following reading:

The vitamins that are needed, as indicated, are contained in Codiron [no longer available] *and* the oil that will counteract the excess of [vitamin] D and produce a *better* regeneration of the activities of the system—it would be very good for everyone where there is a period close to the menopause, or adjustments of any nature—[wheat] germ oil.   538-53

We would begin the wheat germ oil now in small quantities; that is, one minim [drop], increasing one minim daily until ten minims are being taken; then leave off five days, then begin with the one minim again, and so on, see? This will add to the abilities for strengthening the activity of the nerve and muscular forces.   849-44

Again we would add, now the wheat germ oil; not more than the system can stand, but that which aids the natural sources of supplying those energies builded in the system...   849-53

Use of the liquid rather than the capsules is preferred, since, according to the readings, it acts more effectively with the system:

. . .if the wheat germ oil would be taken two drops daily it would be more effective than that prepared in the gelatin capsules; though, to be sure, this may be more convenient to some in the pellets or capsule—but it is not always as fresh, and neither does it act as effectively with the body as being assimilated first with the upper gastric flow.   1158-36

For more details, see appropriate CF.

WHITE'S CODLIVER OIL TABLETS

White's Codliver Oil tablets are a natural source of vitamins A and D, and were recommended in about 50 readings, primarily for body and blood building, in cases such as general debilitation, anemia, poor assimilations, baby care and tendencies toward tuberculosis.

General Debilitation:

Those that will aid in the replenishing of those forces as make for the creating of more red blood, more plasm, through the releasing of the vitamins necessary to make resistance and the activities of the functioning organs near normal, assisting in increasing the weight, these we would continue—in the White's Codliver Oil tablets. Take one or two after each meal.
313-4

. . .the activities of the White's tablets are to make for not only a better activity of the thyroids and the glandular forces in the digestive system but to aid in an appetite.
Do not let either the Ventriculin or the Codliver Oil tablets become so as to replace food values for the system, but be consistent with those things.   528-13

Anemia:

Q-5. What can I do to build up my blood?
A-5. . . .As a tonic for the body. . .we would give rather the White's Codliver Oil tablets, see?   1688-1

. . .if there will be added the thyroids and the beef juices, or the White's Codliver Oil tablets, these would carry the vitamins and sufficient of the iron's creations for the food value, better than iron taken in the system.   773-4

Incoordination Between Assimilations and Eliminations:

. . .these [Codliver Oil tablets] will act—as we find—with the assimilations in such a way and manner as to be less affecting

121

the heart in the circulation with those properties that are being taken for the aiding of the circulation in the present.

3833-1

In a reading for a child, indexed under "body building," the Cayce source advised the taking of the White's tablets in cycles:

These may be taken once a day for a period of a week to two weeks, and then left off for a little while. We will find, or the individuals will find, administering these: To take continually grows not only monotonous to the developing body but if these are taken for periods, let the body adjust itself for a period of a week or ten days to two weeks, and then begin again, their reaction upon the system is much more satisfactory. 1206-3

And, in a reading for an individual with toxemia, the Cayce source made some interesting comments:

These [White's tablets] will carry more of the vitamins necessary to supply the blood, that as will make for oxygen in the system; also will clarify the tissue that is sore through the lungs, and working well with the digestive system. 5672-1

WYETH'S BEEF, IRON & WINE

Beef, Iron & Wine is a generic name for a tonic preparation used as a blood and body builder. The beef extract, iron supplement and red wine it contains has a stimulating effect on the system. The Cayce source recommended this combination in over 50 readings in cases of anemia, general debilitation, and other conditions where a building of resistance was needed. The brand most often specified by the readings was Wyeth's, manufactured since around 1883. Although Wyeth's is no longer available, there are many other versions on the market.

ZILATONE

Zilatone is a laxative compound, indicated in about 80 readings for inadequate eliminations and related problems, such as cholecystitis, incoordination between eliminating functions, toxemia, and cases in which the liver needed stimulating. Its ingredients are: bile extract (73 mg.); cascara sagrada, an herbal cathartic (49 mg.); pancreatin, used for its enzymatic action in various forms of digestive failure (40 mg.);

phenolphthalein (32 mg.); pepsin, 1 to 10,000 (10 mg.); and capsicum (a carminative). The manufacturers report no known changes in this formula since Cayce's day. It is interesting that several readings mention that Zilatone contains a mild heart stimulant but did not say which ingredient was referred to [perhaps Capsicum?]. The readings comment on the use of Zilatone as follows:

Have those regular periods when the Zilatone is used for assisting in creating a better activity through the liver area itself, when there arise any distasteful conditions from the gastric forces of the body itself. Use same periodically then. No activity of such a nature should be used continuously, to be sure, but let the *system* react and then we may have the *proper* reaction from such properties as are combined in such preparations.   1140-2

The readings sometimes commented that Zilatone was superior to some other laxative compounds because it put less strain on the system:

. . .these are a combination of the bile salts as well as the active forces that work with the secretions of the liver itself. But they do not *strain* the system as some of the cathartics that are taken.   1196-1

For while the Zilatone [tablets] carry as an active principle those that are of the nature that arise from the ingredient that is a derivative of senna and of Dovers' Powders, they are not as severe—and make for a more *concerted* action in the direct functioning of the liver *as* it is related to the gall duct area, and not as severe upon the aorta artery circulation or that between the liver and the heart. And they carry a little heart stimulant.
                                          760-20

It was sometimes stressed that while Zilatone was being taken there should be a minimum of physical activity to enable the cleansing elements in the Zilatone to work with the system more efficiently:

We would use Zilatone tablets as a stimuli for the draining of the gall duct area; stimulating activity through the liver as related to the duodenum; stimulating activities of the digestive forces—due to the quietude or lack of physical activity of the body.   533-9

Zilatone was frequently recommended in combination with

Fleet's Phospho-Soda in a procedure designed specifically to drain the gall duct. For details regarding this procedure, the readings should be consulted.

The readings persistently advise the drinking of large quantities of water during the time the Zilatone is taken:

Zilatone is an active force with the liver, pancreas and spleen, and aids in the digestive forces—providing quantities of water are taken at the time.   **533-10**

Finally, as with any laxative, the use of Zilatone should not be continued day after day after normal conditions have been established, but only occasionally when there is need of such a stimulant:

As we find in the present, then, there are these needs: that there be not too often taken those properties [Zilatone] that have been given to work with the gastric flow—by causing or producing an emptying of the gall duct itself. If this is continued to be done, we only *drain* the system without eliminating properly through the system or allowing it to become properly balanced.

We would use then the enemas, rather than taking so much of the Zilatone. However, at times it may be necessary to take the Zilatone for the stirring of the liver; once a week, once in two weeks or once a month, to stir the liver, the pancreas and the spleen and the gall duct area. If there is a feeling of heaviness, a little dizziness, it is very well to take same—but do not continue to take it day after day, day after day and day after day, and then expect it to get the body properly balanced.

     1196-5

A possible substitute for Zilatone might be Caroid Laxative. Some of the ingredients are the same. Caroid Laxative, formerly called Caroid and Bile Salts Tablets, was recommended in the readings before Zilatone came on the market and for some time afterward.

For more information, see the CFs on Intestines: Constipation and Stomach: Indigestion.

It is recommended that you consult a physician before using this product.

INDEX

acidity 2, 7, 48
Acigest 1
Acne Scar Massage 1
acne 1, 8, 9, 41, 62, 64, 102
Adiron 1
adrenalin 12
adrenals 40, 53, 55
agar 72
aging 46
Al-Caroid 2, 7, 18
alcohol
  beverage 30, 60, 116
  grain 38, 40, 42, 48, 52, 56, 57, 61,
    71, 80, 87, 89, 95, 100
  rubbing 52
alcoholism, treatment 60
alkalizer 31
allergies 57
Alpine Ray/Rino Ray 2
ambergris 28, 30
ambrosia weed, see *ragweed*
anemia 1, 36, 77, 90, 113, 121, 122
  pernicious 108
antacid 2, 7, 79
Anti-Nausea Formula 2
antiseptic 1, 26, 67, 106
  intestinal 58, 66
appendicitis 21, 95
appetite 29
apple diet 22, 103
Armour's Liver Extract 52
arteriosclerosis 10
arthritis 3, 4, 6, 15, 21, 77, 80, 89, 100,
  113, 120
Arthritis Massage Formula 3
artichokes, Jerusalem 29, 76
assimilations 21, 26, 38, 48, 76, 82
  poor 1, 2, 14, 36-37, 49, 60, 77, 78, 121
  incoordination with eliminations
    2, 17, 21, 28, 45, 48, 98, 121
asthma 6, 11, 68
astringent 1, 10, 37
athlete's foot 4, 44, 97
Athlete's Foot Remedy 4, 44
Atomidine 4, 33, 41, 52, 53, 60, 90,
  104, 108, 113, 119
attitude 82
Ayurveda 73

baby care 9, 23, 31, 32, 74, 79, 105, 122
  nausea 2
  diaper rash 57
backache 85
baking soda 20, 21, 66
baldness 5, 39, 44, 61, 87, 100, 114

Balm of Gilead 64
balsam
  Canadian 71
  of sulphur 6
  of tolu 9, 47, 64, 71, 95
  Peruvian 9
Battle Creek Sanitorium 25
B-Battery 6
bedbug juice, see *Cimex lectularius*
bedsores 67, 73
benzoin, tincture of 16, 36, 71, 85
  acid 44
Benzosol 7
bicarbonate of soda 7, 60, 101
  rinsing agent 6
bile
  extract 122
  salts 17
birth injuries 10
Bisodol 2, 7
bites 42, 57
Black & White Products 8
black haw 51
blackheads 10
black root 78
bladder 31, 104, 118
blindness 93
blood 64, 77, 121, 122
  pressure 47, 66, 78
  purifier 55, 65, 112
blue 54
body powder 9
boils 6, 64, 73, 104, 105
boncilla packs 9
bones
  chicken 14
  diseases 36
brain damage (in children) 33
brandy, apple 25
breasts 33
bromide of soda 60
bronchitis 11, 68
bruises 73, 85
buchu leaves 47
bunions 21, 101
burdock 47, 51
burns 16, 19, 99
bursa 15

caecum 22
calamus oil 10
Calcidin 5, 11
Calcios 5, 14, 79
calcium 11, 14
  calcium chloride 73

125

READINGS DIRECTORY

786-2	23	1158-38	88	1800-34	73
808-3	39	1165-1	16	1807-3	58
808-8	70	1173-1	108	1842-1	54
811-4	8	1179-1	108	1844-2	92
813-2	117	1179-3	21	1861-11	117
816-1	29, 40	1196-1	123	1968-3	109
826-1	62, 69	1196-5	124	1968-7	10, 20, 78, 80
826-3	90	1196-9	47	1981-1	54
837-1	69	1196-17	114	2015-4	32
839-1	55	1200-6	17	2015-6	16
843-2	66-67	1206-3	122	2015-10	78, 99
843-6	84	1206-13	3	2036-6	36, 37
849-43	15	1206-15	33-34	2048-8	118
849-44	120	1208-3	15	2051-1	18
849-46	43	1208-5	20	2072-6	8, 20
849-53	120	1208-9	72	2072-14	88
849-63	72	1208-16	104	2072-16	10
850-2	41, 62	1247-1	100	2085-1	54, 55
852-13	87	1278-1	56	2096-2	92
856-1	109	1299-1	48	2132-1	54
861-1	88	1312-3	21	2153-5	82
877-18	92	1315-1	112	2153-6	81-82
888-1	113	1419-3	99	2154-2	8, 109
903-16	70	1422-1	29	2168	14
916-1	38	1431-2	87	2175-2	8
916-2	38	1433-6	20	2176-1	24-25
928-1	79	1521-2	5	2180-1	109
934-2	71	1521-4	13	2186-1	67
951	14	1540-3	112	2190-1	50
951-7	15, 118	1541-5	43	2207-1	88
953-1	28	1541-6	84	2289-1	32
953-26	29	1548-4	14, 26	2315-1	101
954-2	13	1553-7	22	2332-1	31
957-3	91	1553-20	114	2341-1	103
970-1	87	1554-27	27	2344-5	90
979-3	113	1557-1	26	2434-3	22
984-5	97	1560-1	12	2448-1	26
985-1	18	1572-1	116	2452-2	46
987-1	74	1573-2	42	2455-1	103
1001-10	83	1584-1	112	2462-3	103
1012-1	39, 65	1596	14	2474-1	48
1019-1	39, 56	1611-2	111	2509-1	100
1022-1	91	1688-1	121	2514-7	67
1026-1	75	1688-7	80	2518-1	97
1034-1	21	1695-2	118	2521-1	21
1045-10	12	1702-1	43	2528-4	114
1057-1	18	1709-4	10	2548-1	63
1100-6	48	1709-5	10	2646-6	94
1100-17	29	1711-1	102, 104	2674	103
1101-4	76	1739-1	29	2680-1	33
1110-4	13	1745-4	59	2752-3	79
1120-2	114	1770-4	101	2768-1	78
1131-2	71	1792	14	2781-1	9
1140-2	123	1800-1	76	2781-2	32-33
1141-1	17	1800-5	92	2790-1	63, 65
1148-1	118	1800-16	92	2790-3	115
1158-31	3	1800-20	106	2803	103
1158-36	120-121	1800-25	119-120	2834-2	56

2843-4	102	3594-1	26	5000-2	56
2946-1	109	3598-1	74	5004-1	11
2975-1	69	3620-1	97	5016-1	101
2998-3	71	3678-1	103	5037-1	84
3033-1	88	3696-1	75	5038-1	33
3050-2	58	3722-1	29	5053-1	26
3051-3	8, 35	3738-1	11-12	5057-1	54, 56, 57
3060-1	117	3776-13	101	5097-1	31, 58
3075-1	116	3810-1	51	5121-1	75
3094-1	70	3833-1	121-122	5148-1	83
3104-1	58	3902-1	76	5178-1	56
3107-1	70	3987-1	70	5188-1	34
3109-1	31, 97-98	4049-1	100	5215-1	56
3157-1	59	4056-1	44	5237-1	56
3158-2	116	4101-1	46	5261-1	89, 97
3160-1	22	4253-1	117	5280-1	56
3176-1	26	4288-1	47	5339-1	114
3180-1	70	4332-1	29	5347-1	96
3246	35	4414-2	29	5450-3	64
3261	103	4510-1	98	5467-1	86
3304-1	4	4581-1	61	5480-1	28, 30
3326-1	24	4678-1	82	5514-3	27
3363-1	3, 78	4735-1	93-94	5545-1	99
3379-1	87	4831-2	111	5566-5	107
3416-1	54	4843-1	116	5640-1	115
3517-1	86	4844-3	80	5672-1	122
3572-1	28	4873-1	106	5676	30
3574-1	18	4874-1	70	5707-1	29

MEDICAL FILES-Alphabetical Listing

Medical files are not for sale. Suggested treatments for any particular ailment should not be "lifted" from any individual reading and tried by another individual except under the supervision of a doctor or other licensed physician. Names of referral doctors will be supplied to members on request. *Numbered volumes count as separate files.*

*File contains commentary or summary by a doctor.

†A physician's notebook is available with the file.

Abdominal Hernia
Abnormal Children
Abnormal Menstruation
Abscessed Ears
*Acidity-Alkalinity
*Acne
Alcoholism, Vols. 1-3
*Allergies: General
*Almonds
Alzheimer's Disease
*Amyotrophic Lateral Sclerosis
*Anemia
*Angina Pectoris
*Aphonia
*Apoplexy
Appendicitis
Applicances: Radio-Active
  (Impedance Device)
  Wet Cell
*Arteriosclerosis
*Arthritis, Vols. 1-4
Asthenia
*Asthma
*Athlete's Foot

Baby Care (See topical list)
*Baldness, Vols. 1 & 2
Bedsores
Bedwetting
Bladder: Stricture
Blepharitis
Blindness, Vols. 1-3
Blindness: Tendencies
Boils, Vols. 1 & 2
Brain Tumors
Breast Cancer
Breast Tumors
Bright's Disease

Bronchiectasis
*Bronchitis, Vols. 1 & 2
Burns: General
*Bursitis

Callouses
Cancer: General, Vols. 1 & 2
Cancer: Lymphosarcoma
Cancer of Face and Throat
Cancer of Stomach and Intestines,
  Vols. 1 & 2
Canker Sores
Carbuncles
*Castor Oil Packs
*Cataracts
Catarrh: Nasal (Rhinitis)
Cerebral Palsy, Vols. 1 & 2
Cerebral Palsy, Abnormal
  Children
Child Training: Behavioral
  Problems
Children: Abnormal: Spiritual
  Healing
Chorea (St. Vitus Dance)
Circulation, Poor
Cirrhosis
*Colds: Coryza
*Colitis
Colitis: Ulcerative
Colon: Impaction, Vols. 1 & 2
*Color Blindness
Complexion
*Constipation
Coronary Thrombosis
*Cystitis
Cysts: General, Vols. 1 & 2
Cysts: Skin

Deafness: Nerve
Deafness: Prolapsed Eustachian
  Tube, Vols. 1-3
Dentistry
Depression (Melancholia), Vols. 1-3
Dermatitis
Detached Retina
*Diabetes, Vols. 1-3
Diarrhea
Disks
*Diverticulitis
Dropsy (Edema, Ascites)
  *Duodenal Ulcers

Eczema
*Emphysema
Encephalitis
Enteritis

135

Poison Ivy
Poliomyelitis
Polycythemia
Possession, Vols. 1-3
Possession: Tendencies
Pregnancy: General, Vols. 1 & 2
Pregnancy: Monthly Sequence
*Prostatitis
Pruritus (Itching), Vols. 1 & 2
*Psoriasis, Vols. 1 & 2
Psychosomatics
Puffy Eyes
Purpura
Pyelitis
*Pyorrhea, Vols. 1 & 2

Raynaud's Disease
Rectal Itching, Vols. 1 & 2
Retinitis Pigmentosa
Rheumatic Fever
Rheumatism
Rheumatism and Neuritis,
    Vols. 1 & 2
Rheumatism: Sciatica
Ringworm

St. Vitus Dance (Chorea)
Sarcoma
Scarlet Fever
*Scars
Schizophrenia, Vols. 1 & 2
Sciatica
†*Scleroderma, Vols. 1 & 2
Scoliosis
Seborrhea
Senility
Serums: Vaccines
Shingles (Herpes Zoster)
*Sinusitis
Skin Cancer
Spine: General
Spine Injuries: Coccyx
Sprains
Sterility: Female
Sterility: Male
Sterility: Tipped Womb
Streptococcus: Infection
Stuttering
Sunburn
*Syphilis: Female
*Syphilis: Male

Tachycardia: Paroxysmal, Vols. 1 & 2
Tic Douloureux
Tinnitus
*Tonsillitis
Torpid Liver
Torticollis

Toxemia, Vols. 1 & 2
Tuberculosis, Vols. 1 & 2
Tumors: General

Ulcers: Skin & Bedsores
*Ulcers: Stomach
Uremia
Uterus: Cancer
Uterus: Tumors

Vaccines
Vaginitis
*Varicose Veins
Vertigo
Vitiligo
von Recklinghausen's Disease

*Warts and Moles
Wilm's Tumors
Whooping Cough

Xeroderma
X-Ray Burns